Anaesthetic Aide-Memoire
2nd Edition

Anaesthetic Aide-Memoire
2nd Edition

Dr John Urquhart
Dr John Hall

with

Dr Pamela Chrispin
Dr Jeremy Mauger
Dr Deborah Meldrum
Dr John Slade

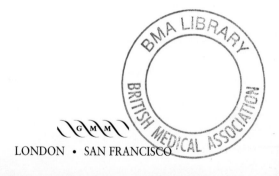

LONDON • SAN FRANCISCO

Typeset by Mizpah Publishing Services, Chennai, India

Printed in the UK by The Cromwell Press

CONTENTS

INTRODUCTION

The *Anaesthetic Aide-Memoire* is a compilation of lists and diagrams intended as a ready reference for senior anaesthetists in training and for consultants in anaesthesia. It is not, and is not meant to be, a definitive pocket textbook of anaesthesia; it is for reference when a fact, statistic, or formula eludes the memory. It is also an aid to teaching.

It covers lists, numerical data, physiological and pharmacological formulae, and information on illnesses pertaining to anaesthesia, data on equipment, clinical measurement, and intensive care management. It includes recent recommendations by the Royal College of Anaesthetists and the Association of Anaesthetists of Great Britain and Ireland, on safety, audit, and other postgraduate matters. It does not include anatomy; there are textbooks on anatomy for anaesthetists. It does not deal with the derivations of physiological and pharmacological equations. Neither is it a pharmacopoeia. This book is intended for anaesthetists who have passed that stage, but who merely want to be reminded of a particular equation or formula prior to using it clinically or asking a junior to produce it in a practice exam.

It will also be useful for candidates for the FRCA Examination, who will already understand the physiology and pharmacology but who need their memory jogged on occasion.

We are indebted to the following people and organisations for their help.

The UK Resuscitation Council for permitting the use of their algorithms.

The Early Warning Score was first developed by Dr Maggie Wright of James Paget Hospital Great Yarmouth. We thank her for permission to publish her work and for help with editing.

The acute pain pages are based on the work of the following: Jessica Atherton and Christine Waters, Acute Pain Service

West Suffolk Hospital, Sara Kinna and Rhea Sapsford, Acute Pain Service Addenbrooke's Hospital and the Pain Service at Queens Medical Centre Nottingham. Thank you for permitting us to use your work in this book.

John Urquhart and John Hall

Bury St Edmunds, March 2004

LIST OF ABBREVIATIONS

AF	Atrial fibrillation
ALA	Aminolaevulinic acid
ALT	Alanine aminotransferase
AP	Action potential
ARDS	Acute respiratory distress syndrome
ARF	Acute renal failure
ASB	Assisted spontaneous breathing
ASD	Atrial septal defect
AST	Aspartate aminotransferase
BBB	Blood-brain barrier
BIPAP	Biphasic positive airway pressure
BMI	Body mass index
BS	Breath sounds
BSA	Body surface area
BSB	Body surface burn
CAVH	Continuous arterio-venous haemofiltration
CEPOD	Confidential enquiry into perioperative deaths
CI	Cardiac index
CPAP	Continuous positive airway pressure
CRF	Chronic renal failure
CRP	C-reactive protein
CSF	Cerebrospinal fluid
CVA	Cerebrovascular accident
CVP	Central venous pressure
CVS	Cardio vascular system
CVVH	Continuous veno-venous haemofiltration
DVT	Deep vein thrombosis
ECG	Electrocardiogram
ESR	Erythrocyte sedimentation rate
F	Frequency of ventilation
FDP	Fibrin degradation products
FGV	Flow generated ventilators

FiO_2	Inspired fraction of oxygen
FRC	Functional residual capacity
GCS	Glasgow coma scale
HD	Haemodialysis
HDU	High-dependency unit
HPF	High-power field
INR	International normalised ratio
IPPV	Intermittent positive pressure ventilation
LAH	Left atrial hypertrophy
LBBB	Left bundle branch block
LMA	Laryngeal mask airway
LMWH	Low molecular weight heparin
LSCS	Lower segment Caesarean section
LVH	Left ventricular hypertrophy
MAC	Minimum alveolar concentration
MAOI	Monoamine oxidase inhibitors
MAP	Mean airway pressure
MH	Malignant hyperpyrexia
MS	Multiple sclerosis
NCEPOD	National CEPOD
ODC	Oxyhaemoglobin dissociation curve
PAN	Polyarteritis nodosa
PAP	Pulmonary artery pressure
PCA	Patient controlled analgesia
PD	Peritoneal dialysis
PDA	Patent ductus arteriosus
PE	Pulmonary embolism
PEEP	Positive end expiratory pressure
PGV	Pressure generated ventilators
PPH	Post partum haemorrhage
PRV	Pressure relief value
PSP	Patient system pressure
PTF	Post-tetanic facilitation
RAH	Right atrial hypertrophy
RBBB	Right bundle branch block
RVH	Right ventricular hypertrophy

SBE	Subacute bacterial endocarditis
SLE	Systemic lupus erythematosus
SVR	Systemic vascular resistance
TIVA	Total intravenous anaesthesia
TPA	Tissue plasminogen activator
U&E	Urea and electrolytes
V_E	Minute ventilation
VE	Ventricular ectopic
VSD	Ventricular septal defect
V_T	Tidal volume
VT	Ventricular tachycardia
#NOF	Fractured neck of femur

THINKING AND TEACHING

Life is too short to drink flat tonic

John Winn

On education:
For most men it remains true and even obvious that for the best education a complete general training in fields other than those of their future calling brings about a richer result.

Bill's observation: That a person may be educated beyond their intelligence.

On anaesthesia and medicine:
You are more likely to die on the first day of your life than on any other than your last.

Prof John Davis

If the surgeon cuts a vessel and knows the name of that vessel, the situation is serious; if the anaesthetist knows the name of that vessel, the situation is irretrievable.

Dr M Morgan

III	At a cardiac arrest the first procedure is to take your own pulse
IV	The patient is the one with the disease
VII	There is no body cavity that cannot be reached with a 14 g needle and a good strong arm
X	If you don't take a temperature you can't find a fever
XIII	The delivery of medical care is to do as much nothing as possible

Samuel Shem

Smith's law of pharmacology: If a drug is lipid soluble, it will be absorbed orally, it will cross the blood-brain barrier (BBB) and the placenta, it will be reabsorbed by the kidneys and will therefore be metabolised and conjugated; if a drug is water soluble, it will not be absorbed orally, it will not cross the BBB or the placenta, and will be filtered by the kidneys.

Extremes of opinion and practice are the posts that mark out the path of medical progress.

Always remember that the kit you are using was made by the lowest bidder.

Salmon's law: When anaesthetising children, the sum of the pulse rate of the child and the anaesthetist will always equal 150.

Winn's modification: That a coefficient be applied to Salmon's law where the more junior and frightened the anaesthetist the greater is that coefficient.

Aunty Gwen's rule: Wait until you see upper limb flexion before you take the tube out and you won't see laryngospasm.

Muscle relaxants do not make the hole bigger, they do not relax bone, they do not decompress bowel, they do not give a surgeon judgement, and they do not relax fat.

You can take an orthopaedic surgeon to slaughter, but you can't make him think.

Dr Phil Keep

On making it count:
Sutton's law: Sutton, an American bank robber, was asked as he was about to be hanged, why he robbed banks. 'Because that's where the money is'.

Cullen's law: Rugby is a game of possession, but mostly of territory; in order to win, any incursion beyond the enemy's 22 metre line must result in the scoring of points.

On sex:
The Urquhart-Malyon law: The innuendo implies the deed; in other words, if you see two people

behaving as if they're having it off, they very probably are.

On intensive care:

Thorp's maxim of intensive care: If a patient isn't going forwards, he's going backwards.

The management of an intensive care patient is characterised by an initial period when resuscitation calls for administration of large quantities of fluid, and a subsequent period when it has to be retrieved.

The time to do a laparotomy is when you first think of it.

To a man with a hammer, everything looks like a nail.

Barbara Morgan on obstetrics:

General anaesthesia for Caesarean section for foetal distress kills mothers who had nothing wrong with them.

The anaesthetist is there to look after the mother: The paediatrician is there to look after the baby: The obstetrician is there to look after himself.

The decision regarding surgery is the obstetrician's. The anaesthesia must be left to the anaesthetist.

Seventeen rules of lecturing

1. Don't apologise for having insufficient time
2. Don't apologise for the subject you're presenting
3. Don't turn your back on the audience
4. Don't use grubby, faded, or handwritten visual aids
5. Don't obstruct the view of the screen, with yourself or the projector
6. Don't use abbreviations or acronyms without explaining them
7. Don't use annoying mannerisms
8. Don't invite students to write it down and then snatch the overhead away
9. Don't wave the laser pointer around the screen or the audience

10. Do make sure you know where everything is in the lecture theatre before you start
11. Do introduce yourself
12. Do say at the beginning what you are going to talk about – and what you aren't
13. Do speak up, and to the back of the room
14. Do make eye contact
15. Do produce a handout, which is intelligible
16. Do present a summary at the end
17. Never use any of the following words or expressions:
    - Interactive
    - It's all in the textbooks
    - Group dynamics
    - Learning curve

How to describe a drug

A mnemonic for the description of any drug or preparation.

Pretty Cute Anaesthetists Can Undo Dresses Regardless Of Displeasure Clearly Covering Sister's Expression In Theatre:

- *Presentation:* Tablets, injection, colour
- *Chemical nature:* Draw if appropriate, e.g. volatiles
- *Action:* At receptor level
- *Class:* e.g. Vaughan-Williams
- *Uses:* Stress anaesthetic uses but do not omit those that the rest of the world uses the drug for
- *Dose:* Obvious
- *Route of administration:* Again, obvious, but don't guess; for example, alfentanil only has a licence for i.v. use, whereas fentanyl has a licence for i.v. and i.m.
- *Onset:* Rapid, slow, delayed
- *Duration of action:* Short, medium, long; state the half-life if you know it
- *Contraindications:* Absolute and relative
- *Complications:* These are the serious ones like asystole and agranulocytosis, in contrast to
- *Side effects:* Which are the trivial ones like nausea and vomiting, but these two do overlap

- *Elimination:* Generally hepatic or renal, but remember pulmonary elimination and excretion of drug into breast milk. In general, if a drug is lipid-soluble, it will be absorbed orally, it will cross the BBB and the placenta, it will be reabsorbed by the kidneys and therefore be eliminated by metabolism and conjugation. If a drug is water-soluble, it will not be absorbed orally, will not cross the BBB or placenta, and will be filtered by the kidneys
- *Interactions:* With what, and the effect: Enhancement of one or other
- *The gravid uterus:* See above

How to handle a clinical nightmare at the primary

- Can I get out of giving this anaesthetic?
- Can I get someone else to give this anaesthetic?
- Can I stall by getting a physician to optimise therapy?
- If I must give it, can I have a senior colleague present?
- Can I get out of giving a GA by using a regional or local technique instead?

— The penetrating eye injury is not a surgical emergency, and can wait until starved, and even then can often be done under local anaesthesia

— #NOFs do not have to be done at 03:00 as long as they are done within 48 h

— At the rapid sequence induction, I shall give a predetermined sleep dose of induction agent, at other times I shall titrate to response

— At the rapid sequence induction, I shall give a calculated dose of suxamethonium immediately the patient is asleep; at other times I shall first ensure that I can control the airway

— If I forget suction at the rapid sequence induction I shall not pass the exam

Four quotable papers which have influenced anaesthetic practice

Chassot PG, Delabays A, Spahn DR: Preoperative evaluation of patients with, or at risk of, coronary artery disease

undergoing non-cardiac surgery. *Br J Anaesth* 2002; 89: 747–59.
How to optimize this group of patients.

Brownridge P: Epidural and subarachnoid analgesia for elective caesarean section. *Anaesthesia* 1981; 36: 70.
First paper describing combined spinal epidural analgesia.

Prys-Roberts C: Isolated systolic hypertension: Pressure on the anaesthetist? *Anaesthesia* 2001; 56: 505–10.
Guidance and algorithm for management of hypertensive patients: it's 160/100, since you ask.

Rodgers A, Walker N, Schug S, *et al*: Reduction of postoperative mortality and morbidity with epidural or spinal anaesthesia: Results from overview of randomised trials. *BMJ* 2000; 321: 1493–97.
Metanalysis of 141 trials and 9559 patients. Incontrovertible evidence that neuraxial blockade reduces postoperative mortality and all markers of morbidity.

PREOPERATIVE MANAGEMENT

This is intended to remind the busy anaesthetist of the essential questions and features of examination and preoperative investigation.

History

Previous general anaesthetics
Family history of allergy or adverse reaction. The important ones are malignant hyperpyrexia and suxamethonium apnoea.

Past medical history
General health and systematic review, with special reference to exercise tolerance, orthopnoea and other indicators of ischaemic heart disease.

Specific questions:
- Coryza or productive cough
- Dyspepsia: If so, is there oesophageal reflux?
- Smokes: Anticipate airway irritability in heavy smokers
  The other problems associated with tobacco include:
  - High carboxyhaemoglobin levels, which impair oxygen carriage
  - Ciliary dysfunction
  - Increased secretions
- Bleeding tendencies: Easy bruising is a good discriminator
- Drugs
- Allergies

Examination

- *Teeth:* Loose teeth, false teeth, caps or crowns
- *Mouth:*

Mallampati classification	Wilson grading (jaw protrusion)
I Uvula, complete view	A Lower incisors beyond upper
II Base of uvula only seen	B Edge-to-edge
III Soft palate in view	C Lower cannot come edge-to-edge. Always difficult.
IV Hard palate only	

- *Neck:* For flexion and extension, and for precipitation of vertebro-basilar insufficiency if susceptible
- *Weight*
- *Chest:* Auscultation; blood pressure, heart rate, heart sounds

Investigations

Use a matrix built around haematology, chemistry, X-ray and clinical measurement to remind you:

Serology sickle	XM, Hb	Potassium	Glucose
Clotting	*Haematology*	Chemistry	Liver function
CXR	*Radiology*	*Clinical measurement*	ECG
Cervical spine	Thoracic inlet	FEV1/FVC, PEFR	Echo

The National Institute for Clinical Excellence (NICE) issued clinical guidelines on the use of routine preoperative tests for elective surgery in 2003. The information can be obtained at http://www.nice.org.uk. The surgical grade and American Society of Anaesthetists grade are used in multiple tables to determine what tests to order.

Surgical grades

Grade 1 (minor)	e.g. Excision lesion of skin
Grade 2 (intermediate)	e.g. Hernia repair
Grade 3 (major)	e.g. TURP
Grade 4 (major+)	e.g. Laparotomy
Neurosurgery	Cardiovascular surgery

American Society of Anesthesiologists (ASA) classification

I	No illness
II	Mild
III	Incapacitating illness
IV	Illness which is a constant threat to life
V	The moribund patient submitted for surgery in desperation is added to denote emergency

Day surgery unit selection criteria

Day surgery may account for more than 50% of elective general surgery. There are financial, patient-satisfaction and waiting list imperatives driving the development of day surgery.

These examples are appropriate for day surgery:

- *General surgery:* Laparoscopic cholecystectomy, hernia repair (open or laparoscopic), varicose veins, circumcision, removal skin lesions, sigmoidoscopy, lymph node biopsy
- *Urology:* Cystoscopy, vasectomy, excision epididymal cyst
- *Gynaecology:* Hysteroscopy, laparoscopy (including sterilisation), termination of pregnancy
- *Orthopaedics:* Arthroscopy, change of plaster, release trigger finger
- *Dental:* Conservation, extractions, frenectomy, removal of metal
- *Ear, nose and throat:* Myringotomy, tonsillectomy, polypectomy, examination under anaesthesia

The following are inconsistent with day surgery:

- *Medical:* Ischaemic heart disease, advanced hypertension, congestive cardiac failure, bleeding disorders, diabetes

mellitus, obesity with body mass index (BMI) over 35, muscular disease, poorly controlled epilepsy
- *Surgical and anaesthetic:* Malignant hyperpyrexia susceptibility, previous anaphylactic reaction to anaesthesia. Suxamethonium apnoea is controversial
- *Social:* No transport, telephone or supervision for 24 h

NCEPOD degree of urgency

- *Elective:* At a time to suit both patient and surgeon
- *Scheduled:* Early operation, usually within 3 wks
- *Urgent:* As soon as possible, usually within 24 h
- *Emergency:* Immediate, resuscitation simultaneous with operation

Nil by mouth

Solids and liquids
Adults are traditionally starved 6 h to solids and 3 h to liquids. Children should be starved for shorter periods. The issue becomes irrelevant in an emergency, although it is valuable to know the duration of the interval between last meal and trauma or administration of opiates, since this is more relevant in terms of gastric emptying than the interval between last meal and induction of anaesthesia.

Thromboembolic risk

Prophylaxis if indicated (see below).

Premedication

- Nothing is so useful as the preoperative visit
- *Patient's normal medication* (but not oral hypoglycaemics, oral anticoagulants, and possibly not monoamine oxidase inhibitors)
- *Nothing: Emla cream and a parent;* In the under three, consider augmenting this with oral atropine (0.425 mg or 0.85 mg)

- *Sodium citrate and H₂ antagonists:* Where reflux is a possibility and a rapid sequence induction is planned
- β-*agonists*; or β-*blockers*? Asthma, or ischaemic heart disease?
- *Fluid preload:* If jaundiced, as prophylaxis against the hepatorenal syndrome
- i.v. *Dextrose and insulin:* In diabetes
- *Opiate or benzodiazepine:* For the traditionalist anaesthetist and the anxious patient – but remember the value of the preoperative visit in allaying anxiety

Scoring in assessment

Glasgow coma scale (GCS)

Eyes open:	
Spontaneously	4
To speech	3
To pain	2
Never	1
Best motor response:	
Obeys commands	6
Localises pain	5
Flexion withdrawal	4
Decorticate flexion	3
Decerebrate extension	2
No response	1
Best verbal response:	
Orientated	5
Confused	4
Inappropriate words	3
Incomprehensible sounds	2
Silent	1

Best score = 15; Worst score = 3.
A score of 8 is regarded as coma.

Apache II score

This provides an indicator of performance; it does not predict outcome, although the sickest patients have the highest scores. It is usually calculated by a computer programme, which will ask for parameters to be entered at a keyboard; it is thus not necessary to know the score attached to a particular parameter, although it is useful to have an overview of how the score is calculated.

Acute physiology score

Score 0 (normal) to +4 (high or low abnormal)
- Temperature
- Mean arterial pressure
- Heart rate
- Respiratory rate
- A-aDO2
- Arterial pH
- Serum sodium
- Serum potassium (doubled in acute renal failure)
- Serum creatinine
- Haematocrit
- Leucocytes
- GCS (3–15)
- Age

Chronic health points

Elective postoperative admission.
Emergency, chronic liver disease, central venous system (CVS), RS, Renal disease or immunocompromise.

Goldman cardiac risk index

Factor	Points
Third heart sound or elevated JVP	11
MI within 6 months	10
Rhythm other than sinus rhythm	7
Ventricular ectopics more than 5/min	7
Age over 70	5
Emergency operation	4
Tight aortic stenosis	3
Poor general condition	3
Thoracic/abdominal operation	3

Risk of cardiac death with a score over 25 is 56%. Note that Goldman did not include angina or hypertension; this has been disputed by other authorities.

Lunn and Mushin 1982: incidence of CVS disease

This is useful data to have in mind when dealing with anaesthesia in the elderly; however well the patient may seem, cardiovascular disease will be present in a large number even though it may be covert.

Age 40–50	6%
Age 50–60	23%
Age 60–70	45%
Age >70	100%

Reinfarction during anaesthesia

This occurs on 3rd postoperative day and has 50–70% mortality.

Months since infarct	Steen, 1978 (%)	Rao, 1983 (%)
0–3	35	5
3–6	12	3
>6	5	1

Rao described aggressive, invasive pre- and postoperative therapy, producing greater safety for the patient with the recent myocardial infarction presenting for surgery.

Miller dyspnoea grades (New York Heart Association)

This provides a useful means of quantifying cardiopulmonary function.

0	No breathlessness
1	Can walk any distance, but needs time
2	Breathless at 100 metres
3	Can walk a few metres only
4	Breathless at rest

The electrocardiogram (ECG)

This is a brief aid to analysing the electrocardiogram in a methodical fashion.

- *Name and Age:* Make sure the ECG belongs to the correct patient
- *Gain:* 10 mm/mV
- *Recording rate:* 25 mm/sec is usual, but 50 mm/sec may be used to analyse a tachycardia
- *Rhythm*
- *Heart rate:* Small square (ssq) = 0.04 sec, large square = 0.2 sec: Heart rate = 300/n of large squares
- *Axis:* Using I and aVf as vectors (normal axis is +ve in I and aVf)
- *P waves* should be <3 ssq wide, <2.5 high in II
- *PR interval* should be 0.12–0.2 sec, 3–5 ssq
- *QRS:* Duration should be <3 ssq; look for Q waves, R progression and R & S amplitude
- *ST segments*
- *QT interval:* QT corrected (QTc) = $QT/\sqrt{RR}$ interval (normal QTc <0.44 sec)
- *T waves ?U waves*

Disease patterns on ECG

Hypertrophic conditions

- *Left ventricular hypertrophy (LVH):* Left axis deviation (LAD), tall R in V5,6, deep S in V2; T inversion in I, II, III, V5,6
- *Right ventricular hypertrophy (RVH):* Right axis deviation (RAD), tall R in V1–4, R = S in V5; T inversion V1,2
- *Left atrial hypertrophy (LAH):* Broad notched P
- *Right atrial hypertrophy (RAH):* Tall peaked P

Defects of rhythm

- *Atrial fibrillation (AF):* No P waves, QRS irregularly irregular
- *Atrial flutter:* P rate 300/min, variable conduction
- *Atrial extrasystole:* Abnormal P, normal QRS
- *Nodal extrasystole:* No P, normal QRS

- *Ventricular extrasystole:* No P, abnormal QRS
- *Bigeminy:* Ventricular ectopic (VE) coupled to a normal PQRST
- *Escape:* Nodal ectopic or VE during sinus arrest or brady-cardia
- *Sinus tachycardia:* Rate <150/min
- *Supraventricular tachycardia:* Rate usually >150/min, no P waves; often nodal in origin
- *Broad complex tachycardia:* Usually ventricular in origin (suggested by deep S in V6) or junctional with a bundle branch block (dominant R in V1)
- *Ventricular tachycardia (VT):* Defined as >3 VE in a salvo
- *VF:* Chaos
- *Torsade des pointes:* VT of writhing morphology

Defects of conduction

- *Wolff-Parkinson-White (WPW):* Short PR, δ-wave before QRS
- *First degree atrio-ventricular (A-V) block:* >0.2 sec (5 ssq)
- *Second degree A-V block (Mobitz 2):* Most beats normally conducted, occasional P not followed by QRS
- *Wenckebach A-V block:* Progressive prolongation of PR until non-conduction occurs
- *Third degree (complete) A-V block:* Dissociation of P from QRS
- *Right bundle branch block (RBBB):* QRS > 0.12 sec (3 ssq), RAD, MaRRoW (QRS morphology changes from M shape to W shape across anterior chest leads)
- *Left bundle branch block (LBBB):* QRS > 0.12 sec (3 ssq), WiLLiaM (QRS morphology opposite to RBBB), T inversion
- *Left anterior hemiblock:* QRS > 0.12 sec (3 ssq), LAD

Coronary vascular disorders

- *Myocardial infarction (MI):* ST elevation, Q waves, T inversion in affected leads
- *Ischaemia:* ST depression horizontally, commonly in lateral leads
- *Pericarditis:* ST depression concave upwards, all leads
- *Pulmonary embolism (PE):* S > R in I, Q in III, T inversion in III; RAD

Electrolytes and drugs
- *Hypokalaemia:* Long QT, flat T, U wave
- *Hyperkalaemia:* Tall peaked T
- *Hypocalcaemia:* Long QT
- *Digitalis:* ST down slope, T inversion

Echocardiogram
As this becomes more widely available so it becomes more valuable. A valve can be stenosed, normal or regurgitant; the left ventricle can be good, moderately impaired or severely impaired, based on ejection fraction (see Physiology). Beware aortic stenosis and particularly if the gradient is >30 mmHg.

The chest X-ray

- *Name, labelled side:* The name may reveal that the patient is at particular risk of, for example, pulmonary tuberculosis; The age is relevant in interpretation of pathological changes
- *P-A or A-P:* The latter are often portable films, taken in accident and emergency or intensive care, and evaluation of the heart size may be inappropriate
- *Hardware:* Endotracheal tube, central venous cannulae, drains
- *Rotation:* From position of clavicles in relation to vertebral column
- *Penetration:* It should be possible to define thoracic vertebrae with correct penetration
- *Soft tissues:* Breasts, surgical emphysema
- *Bony skeleton:* Ribs, spine; metastatic diseases, fractures
- *Trachea:* Size, deviation in malignant disease or pneumothorax
- *Upper mediastinum:* Loss of definition indicates collapse of adjacent lobe. Increased diameter suggests vascular trauma
- *Lung fields:* Pneumothorax, fluid, vessels; Increased density with loss of volume is collapse, increased density without loss of volume implies consolidation
- *Hila:* Position, fissures

- *Diaphragm:* Costo-phrenic angles, for effusions, gas beneath in perforated viscus
- *Heart and aorta:* Loss of definition indicates collapse of adjacent lobe
- *Hidden areas:* Behind diaphragm and heart, apices

Arterial blood gases

When examining a blood gas result, it is wise to be methodical.
1. $PaCO_2$ is related to ventilatory status
2. Consider pH in context of $PaCO_2$ (see below)
3. PaO_2 with inspired O_2 fraction implies hypoxic status

Only a certain number of combinations exist, and diagnosis can be based on three patterns of ventilation; low, normal or high $PaCO_2$.

$$pH \propto \frac{HCO_3}{CO_2}$$

Alveolar hyperventilation: PaCO₂ <3.8 kPa
a. pH >7.5   Acute hyperventilation
b. p H 7.4–7.5   Chronic hyperventilation
c. pH 7.3–7.4   Partly compensated metabolic acidosis
d. pH <7.3   Metabolic acidosis

Normal ventilation: PaCO₂ 3.8 −6.8 kpa
a. pH >7.5   Acute metabolic alkalosis
b. pH <7.3   Acute metabolic acidosis

Respiratory failure: PaCO₂ >6.8 kpa
a. pH >7.5   Partly compensated metabolic alkalosis
b. pH 7.3–7.5   Chronic ventilatory failure
c. pH <7.3   Acute ventilatory failure

Nunn 1988 Northwick park

This was a paper describing 42 cases of severe respiratory disease presenting for surgery, all having general anaesthesia. They all had FEV1 less than 1.0 litre. Only 4 of the 42 required postoperative ventilation.

The conclusion is that best predictors of requirement for post-operative ventilation are:

- PaO_2 <7.2 kPa
- Dyspnoea at rest

Anaesthesia 1988: 43; 543–51.

Simplified Davenport diagram

Simplified to the level that can be recreated on the back of an envelope and in an exam, but remaining useful.

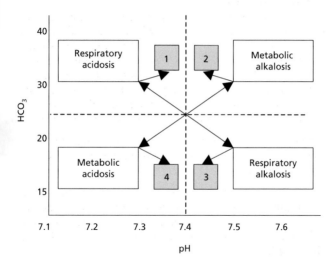

Compensation occurs towards the 7.4 line, i.e. renal H^+ excretion and HCO_3 retention as shown.

1 = Renal (metabolic) compensation for respiratory acidosis.
2 = Respiratory compensation for metabolic alkalosis.
3 = Renal (metabolic) compensation for respiratory alkalosis.
4 = Respiratory compensation for metabolic acidosis.

Respiratory correction depends on increasing or decreasing minute volume and happens rapidly, over the course of a few minutes. Renal correction depends on bicarbonate retention by the kidney and is a chronic phenomenon, taking hours to days to happen.

Haemoglobinopathies

These are disorders of haemoglobin synthesis. The important distinction is between sickle cell disease, which is a qualitative defect, and thalassaemia, which is a group of quantitative disorders.

Sickle cell disease

Sickle cell disease is acquired by autosomal dominant inheritance, and is found in the Afro-Caribbean and Mediterranean populations. The β-chain of HbA has valine substituted for glutamine at position 6. Heterozygotes are at risk of pulmonary infarcts but protected against malaria. Symptoms in homozygotes occur as acute pain in chest, bone (especially of the femoral head), abdomen, and over the spleen; there may also be cerebrovascular accident or myocardial infarction.

Precipitants include: Hypoxia, acidosis, dehydration, hypothermia, and the use of tourniquets. Homozygotes rarely survive beyond age 50.

Diagnosis: Sickledex test: The reagent is Na metabisulphite. Electrophoresis is then required to distinguish sickle cell trait from sickle cell disease. Exchange transfusion is indicated if HbA is less 40% of haemoglobin, or if total Hb <10 g/dl.

Thalassaemia

This results in a partial (heterozygous, thalassaemia minor) or a complete (homozygous, thalassaemia major) abnormality in the α-chain or β-chain of haemoglobin. α-thalassaemia, because the α-chain is universal to all Hb, is fatal in the major form. β-thalassaemia is the commonest.

As well as these two, there are as many as 100 other haemoglobinopathies which may exist alone or in combination with the above. The commonest of these is HbSC.

Paediatric illnesses

These notes are intended to jog the memory when called to see a condition which you may not have seen in your recent practice.

Pyloric stenosis

The incidence is 1:350, of whom 85% are male. There is a $\downarrow K^+$, $\downarrow Cl^-$ alkalosis with paradoxical urinary excretion of H^+ to maintain Na^+; resuscitation takes priority over surgery.

$$\text{Fluid required for correction (ml)}$$
$$= 2/3 \text{ body weight} \times (106 - [Cl])$$

Methods:
1. Rapid sequence induction
2. Gas induction
3. Awake intubation
4. Local

Tracheoesophageal fistula

The incidence is 1:3,500, males affected equally with females. 85% have a blind oesophageal pouch with fistula distal to trachea. An awake intubation is usual, situating a plain oral tracheal tube distal to the fistula.

Congenital diaphragmatic hernia

The incidence is 1:5,000; females are twice as commonly affected as males. 80% are left sided (Foramen of Bochdalek). 20% also have a cardiovascular defect. Only 50% survive, those with accompanying pulmonary dysplasia doing worse.

Omphalocoele

The incidence is 1:5,000. It is a persistence of the herniation of the gut into the extra-embryonic part of the umbilical cord. The gut is covered by a membrane. Other defects are associated.

Gastroschisis

The incidence of this condition is 1:30,000. This is an ischaemic defect of the anterior abdominal wall, with prolapse of the gut through the defect; the gut is not covered. There are no associations.

Congenital heart defects

These are generally seen in females more than in males, and can be divided into those lesions associated with cyanosis and those not.

Acyanotic	Cyanotic
Ventricular septal defect (VSD)	Transposition of the great vessels
Atrial septal defect (ASD)	Tetralogy of fallot
Patent ductus arteriosus (PDA)	Eisenmengers (a late consequence of prolonged left to right shunt with eventual reversal of pressures)
Pulmonary stenosis	
Aortic stenosis	
Coarctation of the aorta	
Hypoplastic heart	

'Left to right, pink and mighty; right to left, blue and unsightly'

If a shunt goes left to right, effort is wasted and hypertrophy occurs; if a shunt goes right to left, deoxygenated blood is pumped into the systemic circulation and cyanosis occurs.

VSD: This is the commonest congenital cardiovascular lesion seen in neonates. It is characterised by a pansystolic murmur at the left sternal edge and biventricular hypertrophy.

ASD: This may present in the adult; features are an ejection systolic murmur in the pulmonary area, a fixed split second heart sound, and right ventricular hypertrophy.

PDA: There is a continuous murmur in the pulmonary area, and left ventricular hypertrophy.

Coarctation: The classic sign is a pansystolic murmur, radiating to the back. Chest X-ray may show rib notching due to engorged collateral circulation. There will be left ventricular hypertrophy.

Cystic fibrosis

The incidence is 1:2,000 many of whom now reach adulthood. The inheritance is autosomal recessive, with 1:25 carrying the gene, which is on chromosome 7, where more than 200 mutations have been recorded. The underlying defect is of abnormal epithelial chloride and sodium transport resulting in increased electrolyte content of secretions. Presentation is by meconium ileus or, in later childhood, recurrent chest infections (chest illness or heart disease are the cause of death in 95% of affected adults) or malabsorption. Diagnosis is by pilocarpine iontophoresis.

Indications for surgery include bowel surgery in the neonate, polypectomy, or vascular access in childhood, and transplantation in the adult. Active chest infection should be excluded before elective surgery. Electrolyte disturbance (hypokalaemia and hypochloraemia) should be corrected. Desaturation occurs readily and securing the airway by intubation and ventilation is usual. A volatile is useful for bronchodilation. Regional anaesthesia is helpful in the postoperative period for aiding physiotherapy.

Connective tissue diseases

Although these conditions are common and of considerable clinical significance to the anaesthetist, they are over-represented in examinations.

Consider: Under each condition, think about the patient, and the anaesthetic.

Patient: Condition and operation type which may be associated with the condition, for example, arthroplasty in rheumatoid arthritis.

Systems: Effects of the condition on the cardiovascular, respiratory, musculoskeletal, renal, and central nervous systems. Remember the use of drugs.

Anaesthesia: Operation, premedication, induction, airway control, postoperative management. Cervical collars. Deep vein thrombosis and pulmonary embolus prophylaxis.

Diagnosis of connective tissue disease

Erythrocyte sedimentation rate (ESR); rheumatoid factor; antinuclear factor; biopsies of muscle, temporal artery, and kidney.

Rheumatoid

Seen from age 30, eventually affecting 1% population, and 3:1 female to male. There is a 10% association with pericarditis. Anaemia of chronic disease is almost universal. 2% will have fibrosing alveolitis and decreased lung compliance. Peptic ulceration is common. 25% will have occipito-atlanto-axial joint X-ray changes, but only 6% will have symptoms. Anticipate a difficult view of the airway; 53% in one series were Cormack and Lehane grade 3 or 4. The use of steroids is common.

Scleroderma

This is a disease of the middle-aged. It is associated with pulmonary fibrosis, achalasia, polymyositis, and renal failure. The multisystem manifestations of the disease therefore present considerable challenges to the anaesthetist.

Systemic lupus erythematosus (SLE)

The incidence is 1:10,000, with a sex difference of 8:1 female to male. There may be pericarditis, mitral endocarditis (Libman-Sacks), pulmonary fibrosis, and nephrotic syndrome. The use of steroids is common.

Polyarteritis nodosa

Males and females are equally affected. The features are hypertension, asthma, nephrotic syndrome, infarcts and cerebrovascular accidents. Steroids are usually prescribed.

Neurological diseases

Epilepsy: Avoid methohexitone and enflurane, both of which are epileptogenic.

Bells palsy: This is a lower motor neurone lesion and affects the upper part of the face as well as the lower part, in contrast to an upper motor neurone lesion, which will spare the upper part.

Horner's syndrome: This is a sympathetic lesion; everything gets smaller or contracts; the features are therefore a small pupil (miosis), enopthalmos, anhidrosis, ptosis, stuffy nose and flushed skin. It may be associated with a high regional block or with malignant disease (Pancoast tumour of the apex of the lung).

III Nerve palsy: This produces ptosis with an enlarged pupil (mydriasis).

Tentorial coning: This produces 3rd cranial nerve palsy, ↓HR, ↑BP, ↓GCS.

Medullary coning: Associated with ↓respiratory rate and neck stiffness.

Hydrocephalus: Cerebrospinal fluid (CSF) production is 0.3 ml/min in adult, from choroid plexus in the lateral and 3rd ventricles. The total volume is 120 ml and turnover takes place every 4–6 h. CSF is absorbed from arachnoid villi in proportion to the difference between CSF pressure and CVP. In children, it may be associated with spina bifida, from a congenital aqueduct stenosis, or as a result of intracranial bleeding or infection.

Bulbar palsies: The significance of these is that they represent a hazard to airway safety; they fall into two groups:

	Pseudobulbar palsy	Bulbar palsy
Cause	Cerebrovascular accident, multiple sclerosis	Motor neurone disease, Guillain-Barre syndrome
Feature	*Upper* motor neurone lesion	*Lower* motor neurone lesion
Emotion	Labile	Normal
Tongue	Spastic	Fasciculating
Jaw jerk	Increased	Absent

Muscular diseases

Multiple sclerosis (MS): The incidence is 50:100,000. An environmental cause is suspected from the geographical variation in the condition. Diagnosis is made by magnetic resonance imaging. Of those that present with optic neuritis, 50% progress to MS. Symptoms worsen with stress and heat. Suxamethonium causes greater than usual K^+ release. Regional techniques are acceptable, but carry a theoretical risk of accelerating demyelination.

Muscular dystrophies: Cardiac muscle is involved. Suxamethonium causes extreme K^+ release. Patients are more than usually sensitive to non-depolarising neuromuscular blockers.

Myotonia dystrophica: This is a disease transmitted by autosomal dominant inheritance. The features are of wasting, balding, cataracts, diabetes mellitus, and intraventricular conduction defects. Suxamethonium causes excessive K^+ release, and intense myotonia (which can also be caused by neostigmine). Local anaesthetics and regional blocks cause prolonged weakness, including uterine atony. The safe anaesthetic includes propofol, non-depolarising muscle blockers, and opiates. Neostigmine is not safe.

Guillain-Barre: This is an acute postinfective polyneuropathy; it occurs 7–10 days after an infectious (usually viral) illness, producing an ascending paralysis. Maximum disability occurs at 4 wks.

Myasthenia gravis: This is characterised by antibodies to postsynaptic acetylcholine receptors, causing weakness of neuromuscular transmission. It is associated with thymoma. Edrophonium reverses weakness for 10 min and is the basis of the diagnostic 'Tensilon test'.

Eaton-Lambert syndrome: A disorder of acetylcholine release, in contrast to myasthenia gravis, which affects the receptor. It is associated with oat cell carcinoma. Muscle function improves with movement, and the Tensilon test is negative, distinguishing it from myasthenia.

Disorders of consciousness

Consciousness has content and level, and conscious behaviour requires:

- Intact cerebral cortex
- Ascending reticular activating system
- Input of sensory or thought processes

Coma: 'Not obeying any commands, not uttering any words, not opening the eyes'.

Locked-in syndrome: This is a disorder of the content of consciousness. Causes are pontine or midbrain cerebrovascular accident (CVA), or tumour. 60% will not survive.

Persistent vegetative state: This is a disorder of the state of consciousness. There is a functional brain stem, with a damaged cortex (reduced blood flow, retarded visual evoked responses). 45% are due to head injury, 40% to CVA.

Brain stem death: This is described as having 2 preconditions, 6 exclusions, and 7 criteria. See below.

Porphyria

There are broadly two groups of porphyria; erythropoetic and hepatic. Anaesthetic drugs do not precipitate erythropoetic forms. The basis of the condition is induction of the small, inducible enzyme δ-aminolaevulinic acid (ALA) synthetase by pregnancy, diet, infection, alcohol, and drugs including steroids and barbiturates. There is then a deficient enzyme further down the synthetic pathway of haem; the resultant accumulation of small intermediates crossing the blood-brain barrier, cause psychological manifestations; larger ones do not, and cause cutaneous manifestations instead.

Acute intermittent porphyria: Seen in Scandinavia, causing psychosis, defect is protoporphyrinogen I synthase. Diagnosis is based on finding ALA in urine.

Variegate porphyria: Seen in South Africa, affecting skin; defect is protoporphyrinogen oxidase. Diagnosis from finding porphyrins in stool.

The safe anaesthetic includes propofol, nitrous (but probably not other volatiles), vecuronium, opiates, and domperidone. Local anaesthetics are contentious.

Liver disease

Tests

Excretory function: Bilirubin. If unconjugated, this implies excessive haemolysis or hepatic failure, and the bilirubin will be lipid soluble and enter central nervous system. Only conjugated, water soluble, bilirubin, may appear in urine and the presence of this indicates biliary obstruction.

Cell damage: Indicated by elevated transaminases. Hepatitis causes increase in alanine aminotransferase (ALT) over aspartate aminotransferase (AST); tumour and sepsis cause increase in AST more than ALT. Alcohol characteristically causes elevated γGT.

Cholestasis: This is indicated by elevated alkaline phosphatase.

Synthetic function: This is related to albumin level, and a defect of synthetic function will prolong the prothrombin time.

Scoring in liver disease

Child: Class A-B-C; based on bilirubin, albumin level, presence of ascites, whether there is a neurological disorder, and the nutritional status.

Pugh: Score 4–12; based on bilirubin levels, albumin, prothrombin time, and whether there is encephalopathy. A score less than 6 implies good risk, but over 10 indicates a poor operative risk.

Safe anaesthetic in liver disease

Includes fluid rehydration, avoidance of hypotension and care with regional anaesthesia in case of impaired clotting. Thiopentone, atracurium, and isoflurane are acceptable. The risk is of further liver impairment and of the hepatorenal syndrome.

Renal disease

Tests

For renal plasma flow: PAH clearance. Normal = 625 ml/min.

For glomerular filtration rate: Creatinine clearance. Normal = 125 ml/min. EDTA clearance confirms normal function (prior to transplant) but does not quantify abnormality.

Filtration fraction =
Glomerular filtration rate/Renal plasma flow.

Kidney disease can present in only four ways:
1. Proteinuria; if extreme, this is the nephrotic syndrome
2. Haematuria
3. Uraemia; acute or chronic, with consequences, e.g. hypertension
4. Hypertension

Proteinuria

Exists if elimination of protein in urine exceeds 150 mg/24 h; if more than 5 g/24 h and hypoalbuminaemia is present, this is the nephrotic syndrome.

Causes of Proteinuria
- Pyelonephritis (acute and chronic)
- Glomerulonephritis (acute and chronic)
- Obstructive nephropathy
- Congestive cardiac failure
- Postural
- Diabetes mellitus
- Myeloma
- Nephrotic syndrome, which in turn may be due to:
  - Minimal change glomerulonephritis (80%)
  - Diabetes mellitus
  - SLE
  - Heavy metal poisoning (Fanconi syndrome)

Haematuria

Exists if, in the urine, there is elimination of:
- Erythrocytes 1×10^6 cells/24 h (2 per HPF), or
- Leucocytes 2×10^6 cells/24 h (4 per HPF)

Causes of haematuria
- Calculi
- Tumours: Bladder, kidneys, prostate

- Urinary tract infection
- Trauma
- Acute glomerulonephritis: Acute streptococcal glomerulo-nephritis causes the nephritic syndrome of haematuria and oliguria proceeding to oedema
- Malignant hypertension
- Benign prostatic hypertrophy
- Connective tissue disease: SLE, polyarteritis nodosa (PAN)
- Infective endocarditis
- Anticoagulants

Acute renal failure

This is present when urine output is less than 400 ml/24 h.

Causes of renal failure

- Pre-renal; hypovolaemia, shock
- Post-renal; obstruction
- Renal parenchymal:
  - glomerulonephritis
  - Pregnancy induced hypertension
  - Acute tubular necrosis; a dilute oliguria occurs with high filling pressures. It is often a consequence of acute renal failure, and is often self limiting after up to 3 wks of fluid restriction or dialysis. Recovery is heralded by a diuresis and natriuresis
  - Malignant hypertension
  - Connective tissue disease
  - Septicaemia
  - Disseminated intravascular coagulation
  - Hepatorenal syndrome

Safe anaesthetic in renal disease

Includes thiopentone, atracurium, non-depolarising blockade (suxamethonium may have unpredictable duration of action, although many would advocate a rapid sequence induction), and a volatile. Meticulous attention to renal output is required.

$$\text{Dose in renal failure} = \text{Usual dose} \times \frac{\text{normal } t_{1/2}}{\text{observed } t_{1/2}}$$

Plasma cholinesterase genotypes

An abnormal response to suxamethonium, if due to an abnormal form of plasma cholinesterase, may result in prolongation of action, sometimes for several hours. The management involves maintenance of the airway, supporting ventilation, and sedation until the block wears off. The patient, and first-degree relatives, must then be investigated.

Genotype	Incidence	Response to suxamethonium	DN	FN
EuEu	96%	Normal	80	60
EaEa	1:2,800	Very prolonged	20	20
EuEa	1:25	Slightly prolonged	40–60	45
EfEf	1:154,000	Mod. prolonged	70	30
EsEs	1:100,000	Very prolonged	–	–
EuEf	1:200	Slightly prolonged	75	50
EuEs	1:190	Slightly prolonged	80	60
EaEf	1:20,000	Mod. prolonged	45	35
EsEa	1:29,000	Very prolonged	20	19
EfEs	1:150,000	Mod. prolonged	60	35

DN = dibucaine number; FN = fluoride number. The dibucaine number is the % inhibition of enzyme by dibucaine, 10^{-5} M concentration. Normal inhibition is 80%. A homozygous defect results in an abnormal enzyme with reduced affinity for suxamethonium. This also happens to be resistant to dibucaine inhibition. Fluoride inhibition may also be used to further identify the particular genotype; because there are 4 alleles, there are 10 possible genotypes.

Psychiatric drugs

Monoamine oxidase inhibitors (MAOI)

Direct-acting agents (adrenaline, noradrenaline) have no enhanced effect in the presence of MAOI, since adrenaline and noradrenaline both act post-synaptically, whereas MAOI block intraneuronal breakdown. Indirect acting agents (ephedrine), however, are taken up and displace neurotransmitter and in combination with MAOI can precipitate hypertension and subarachnoid haemorrhage, as can pethidine.

Tricyclic antidepressants

These act by blockade of reuptake, and could present a risk of enhanced effect in the presence of direct-acting vasopressors. Their phenothiazine nucleus also confers an antimuscarinic effect. They are arrhythmogenic, especially in the elderly.

Selective serotonin uptake inhibitors

These are very safe in anaesthesia, but co-administration with MAOI can precipitate a neuroleptic-malignant syndrome like event for which dantrolene may be of use.

Lithium

This enhances the effect of neuromuscular blockers, and induction agents. It also carries a risk of renal damage in hypovolaemia.

Steroids

Adrenocortical insufficiency: This occurs in sepsis, tuberculous adrenalitis (Addison's disease), and the Waterhouse-Friedrickson syndrome (haemorrhage into adrenals). The main concern however is from steroid therapy, whether oral, topical, inhaled, or parenteral, which will suppress the pituitary-adrenal axis. Beware also the depot steroids used for chronic pain and atopy. Endogenous cortisol output is 25 mg/day rising to 500 mg/day in stress, which response may not be possible if adrenal suppression exists. This may precipitate an addisonian crisis, which consists of collapse, hyperkalaemia, hyponatraemia, and hypoglycaemia.

Equivalence
- Hydrocortisone 100 mg
- Prednisolone 25 mg
- Betamethasone 4 mg
- Dexamethasone 4 mg

Replacement: Hydrocortisone 100 mg at induction then reduce from 100 mg qds over three days.

Blood products

All donated blood starts as 450 ml from the donor, with 60 ml additive, cooled to 4°C.

CAPD = citrate, adenine, phosphate, dextrose
SAGM = sodium chloride, adenine, glucose, mannitol

Random blood   64% compatible
ABO cross-match   99.4% compatible
ABO + Rh cross-match   99.8% compatible
Full cross-match   99.95% compatible

Product	Vol. (ml)	Additive	Hct	Life
Whole blood	450	60 ml CAPD	0.45	21 days
Plasma-reduced	350	60 ml CAPD	0.60	21 days
SAGM	200	100 ml SAGM	0.60	45 days
Conc. red cells	200	SAGM	0.80	
Human albumin	450	pasteurised 60°C		
FFP (all factors)	200	stored at −30°C		6 months
Cryoprecipitate (mostly factor 8)	15	stored at −30°C		6 months
Platelets	200 ml increase platelet count by 30,000/dl			3 days

Stored blood has the following characteristics: pH 6.9, K^+ 20 mmol/l, HCO_3 10 mmol/l.

Usual filter aperture is 200 μm. When transfusing platelets, use either special platelet filter, or none at all; ordinary filters will block.

Cardiac valves

For all cases

An echocardiogram is the single most useful investigation, demonstrating the appearance of a valve, the pressure gradient across it, the ejection fraction, and ventricular wall motion and thickening. If on therapy, urea and electrolytes (U&E) are indicated. If cardiovascularly compromised, a pulmonary artery catheter is necessary. A medical opinion may be valuable in order to optimise therapy. Physicians are not allowed to pronounce on the safety or otherwise of anaesthesia nor to recommend any particular technique. Remember endocarditis prophylaxis.

Avoid regional techniques, especially with stenotic lesions. The sympathetic block induced in the presence of a fixed output state will cause a catastrophic fall in blood pressure.

Aortic stenosis

Causes: Calcified bicuspid valve or rheumatic heart disease.

Important signs: Ejection systolic murmur, low pulse pressure, chest pain, left ventricular failure, syncope. Sudden death is a feature of this condition.

Key
- Provide adequate filling pressure
- Maintain systemic vascular resistance (SVR)
- Control heart rate

Mitral stenosis

Causes: Rheumatic heart disease.

Important signs: Mid diastolic murmur, AF, emboli, haemoptysis, right ventricular failure.

Points: Often anticoagulated; may be hypovolaemic from diuretic therapy. An ECG is mandatory to establish rhythm.

Key
- Control ventricular rate and maintain sinus rhythm
- Adequate filling pressure
- Maintain SVR
- Avoid pulmonary vasoconstriction

Aortic incompetence

Causes: Acute, Subacute bacterial endocarditis (SBE), Marfan's; requires emergency aortic valve replacement.

Chronic: Rheumatic heart disease

Important signs: Early diastolic murmur, waterhammer pulse, left ventricular dilation and failure.

Key
- Slight tachycardia is beneficial
- Avoid increasing SVR

Mitral incompetence

Causes: Acute, SBE and post MI; these may need emergency mitral valve replacement.

Chronic: Rheumatic heart disease and LVH.

Important signs: Pansystolic murmur, left ventricular failure, with or without right ventricular failure.

Points: Left ventricular dilatation may lead to LVH and so to LAH with pulmonary oedema and then right ventricular failure.

Key
- Slight tachycardia may be beneficial
- Avoid increasing systemic and pulmonary vascular resistance

Other valvular lesions

Pulmonary stenosis, which is usually congenital, and tricuspid incompetence which is seen in SBE and in drug addicts; an important feature of the latter is the presence of a venous pulsation, which provides a misleading pulse oximetry reading.

How to describe a murmur

Where in cycle/where on precordium/radiation/effect of respiration. RILE: Right sided murmurs loudest in Inspiration, Left sided loudest in Expiration. NB – a murmur may not be due to a valve.

How to describe a pulse

- Rate
- Rhythm
- Volume

- Character
- Tension
- Vessel wall
- Equality

Management of paediatric murmurs

This is a common problem; what to do when confronted by a murmur in a child scheduled for surgery, when there will probably not be time to organise preoperative investigation.

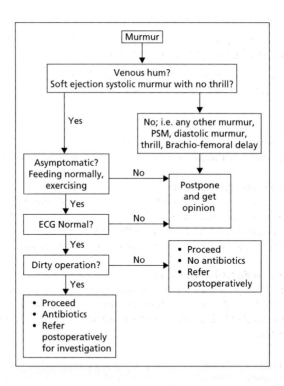

McEwan AI, Birch M, Bingham R: The preoperative management of a child with a heart murmur. *Paediatric Anaesthesia* 1995; 5: 151–6.

Endocarditis prophylaxis

These guidelines change regularly. If in doubt, consult a microbiologist.

Indications: Prosthetic valves, post-SBE (both are at special risk); post-rheumatic fever, mitral regurgitation (MR), mitral stenosis (MS), aortic stenosis (AS), aortic regurgitation (AR), bicuspid aortic valve, ventricular septal defect (VSD), atrial septal defect (ASD), patent ductus arteriosus (PDA). Requirement in mitral leaflet prolapse is controversial.

Dental surgery: Amoxycillin 3 g p.o. 4 h preop (or 1 g i.v. at induction), repeated postop.
- If at special risk: Amoxycillin 1 g + Gentamicin 120 mg i.m. or i.v. at induction, Amoxycillin 500 mg p.o. postop
- If allergic to penicillin, or had a penicillin more than once in last month: Vancomycin 1 g (child, 20 mg/kg) over 100 mins + Gentamicin 120 mg (2 mg/kg) at induction

Urology: As for special risk, above. If infected, appropriate to organism, if identified.

O&G, GI surgery: Only if at special risk: As for urology.

Antithrombotic prophylaxis

Risk groups and incidence of complications
Low risk: <10% deep vein thrombosis (DVT), 0.01% fatal pulmonary embolism (PE)
- Surgery <30 min; no risk factors other than age
- Surgery >30 min; age <40; no other risk factors
- Minor trauma

Moderate risk: 10–40% DVT, 0.1–1% fatal PE
- Major general, urological, gynaecological, cardiothoracic, vascular, neurosurgery; age >40 or other risk factor
- Major trauma, burns
- Minor surgery or trauma with other risk factor

High risk: 40–80% DVT, 1–10% fatal PE
- Surgery of pelvis, hip, lower limb
- Pelvic or abdominal surgery for malignancy

- Major surgery with high risk factors
- Lower limb paralysis
- Amputation

Other risk factors: Obesity, varicose veins, immobility, pregnancy, oestrogens, history of DVT or PE, thrombophilia, malignancy, cardiac disease, connective tissue disease. The Consensus paper on which these guidelines did not, strangely, mention smoking as a risk factor.

Recommendations

- Early mobilisation, all groups
- Specific prophylaxis, moderate and high risk groups
- Continue prophylaxis until discharge

Methods:
- Low molecular weight heparin
- Low dose s/c heparin, 5,000 u 8–12-hourly
- Adjusted low dose s/c heparin, 3,500 u 8-hourly, starting 2 days prior to surgery, keeping APTT upper range of normal
- Warfarin to keep INR between 2.0–2.5
- Dextran 70
- Graduated compression stockings
- Intermittent pneumatic compression
- Anti-platelet drugs, aspirin or hydroxychloroquine

Recommendations by speciality:
General surgery: Medium risk, use low dose heparin or low molecular weight heparin, 12 hourly; high risk, use low dose heparin or low molecular weight heparin, 8 hourly. If contraindicated, then use graduated compression stockings or intermittent pneumatic compression or both.

Urological surgery: Medium risk and high risk use low dose heparin and graduated compression stockings or intermittent pneumatic compression with graduated compression stockings.

Gynaecological surgery: Medium risk use low dose heparin 12 h with graduated compression stockings, or intermittent pneumatic compression with graduated compression stockings. In high risk use low dose heparin 8 h with graduated compression stockings, or intermittent pneumatic compression with graduated compression stockings.

Cardiac surgery: Medium risk and high risk use anti-platelet drugs, either aspirin or hydroxychloroquine.

Vascular surgery: Medium risk and high risk use low dose heparin.

Neurosurgery: Medium risk and high risk use intermittent pneumatic compression with graduated compression stockings.

Orthopaedic:
- Elective hip, medium risk and high risk use low molecular weight heparin or adjusted low dose heparin
- Hip fractures, medium risk and high risk use adjusted low dose heparin or dextran. If cardiac disease present, use warfarin
- Knees, medium risk and high risk use intermittent pneumatic compression with graduated compression stockings

Combined oral contraceptive: If no other risk factors, do not stop oral contraceptive. In emergency or major elective use any method.

Pregnancy: If other risk factor present, low dose heparin (and then onto warfarin) from onset of labour and for 6 wks.

Emergency Caesarean section: If other risk factor present, use low dose heparin until mobile.

From: Thromboembolic risk factors consensus group. *BMJ* 1992; 305: 567–74.

Management of diabetes mellitus

Beware also renal, vascular, and autonomic complications of the disease when considering a diabetic patient.

Preoperative management

The aim is to minimise the metabolic derangement by providing a balance of fluid, calories, and insulin, with care to avoid the hazards, which are:

- Hypoglycaemia
- Hyperglycaemia
- Lipolysis
- Proteolysis
- Ketoacidosis
- Dehydration

The preoperative visit must establish three things:
1. Adequacy of blood sugar control
2. Therapy in use
3. Degree of multisystem involvement

Non-insulin dependant diabetes: minor surgery

- Transfer to short-acting agent one week pre-operatively if possible
- No tablets on morning of operation. Treat as non-diabetic if BS <7 mmol/l
- Restart tablets with first meal
- Give i.v. glucose with caution if at all

Non-insulin dependant diabetes: major surgery

- As for IDDM. See below
- Once eating: tds soluble insulin (Actrapid) 8–12 u before each meal. Revert to tablets once insulin >20 u/day

Insulin-dependant diabetes: Alberti Regime

- Convert to soluble insulin over 3 days
- No insulin in morning of operation
- Set up infusion 500 ml 10% dextrose with 10 u Actrapid and 10 mmol KCl; run at 100 ml/h (adult). Check BS and K^+ every 2 h and adjust as necessary. This entails discarding the entire bag and starting again; this is a major criticism of the regime, as in addition to waste, it makes accurate recording of fluid intake difficult
- Stop infusion when oral feeding recommenced, go to tds Actrapid (Daily dose + 20% if infected, + 20% if on steroids)

Insulin-dependant diabetes: continuous insulin and dextrose

- Convert to soluble insulin
- Commence infusion 10% dextrose from starvation, at 100 ml/h (adult)
- Soluble insulin by infusion; there are a number of 'sliding scales' available

Sönksen P, Sönksen JR. Insulin: Understanding its action in health and disease. *Br J Anaesth* 2000; 85: 69–79.

Obesity

The BMI = weight (kg)/height (m)^2. Normal is 20–25; overweight 25–30, and over 30 is obesity. This is an actuarial index (also known as the Quetelet index) and is used to identify that group which is at greater risk of:

- Hypertension, RVH, ischaemic heart disease and increased oxygen consumption
- Decreased respiratory compliance and reduced functional residual capacity (FRC)
- Gastro-intestinal reflux and hiatus hernia
- Endocrine problems: Glucose tolerance often impaired, sometimes to the point of frank diabetes
- Altered pharmacokinetics: Increased volume of distribution for lipid-soluble drugs, e.g. induction agents

Hypertension

Condition must be optimised and medication must be continued up to and including the morning of operation. Beware co-existing silent ischaemia which occurs in the morning, in the elderly, in diabetics and is three times as common as angina. It is suggested by fatigue, arrhythmia and acute left ventricular failure.

Most would say that a pressure of 160/100 is just acceptable.

A β-blocker e.g. metoprolol 50 mg may be given as a premedicant if the patient is not already on such a drug, as it reduces rate, reduces contractility and is antidysrhythmic.

Critical periods are intubation and extubation, incision and visceral handling, as well as periods of changes in circulating volume. (See also under Initial Assessment, but remember Goldman did not include hypertension in the Cardiac Risk Index).

The hazards confronting the anaesthetist are:	The hazards to the hypertensive patient, greater than to a patient with *controlled* blood pressure, are:
Exaggerated rises in pressure on laryngoscopy and at start of surgery	Stroke on starting anaesthetic (explain difference between 'stroke' and 'heart attack')
Tachycardia and ST segment depression on laryngoscopy and at start of surgery	Heart attack on starting anaesthetic
Sudden hypotensive episodes secondary to alterations in venous return	Stroke during operation
Increased left ventricular wall tension associated with incompliant aortic arch	'Overwork' for the heart
Subendocardial ischaemia during prolonged procedure	Heart attack during operation
Alterations in vascular tone and maldistribution of cardiac output	Damage to liver, kidneys and other organs during operation
Silent postoperative ischaemia and infarction	Heart attack on the ward after operation

MALIGNANCY

Specific problems include:

- Cachexia and poor nutritional state
- Low proteins and enhanced effect of protein-bound drugs.
- Anaemia and cardiac failure
- Hypercalcaemia; levels over 3.75 mmol/l may be reduced by phosphate infusion (or infusion of biphosphonates) in an emergency, or by oral phosphate, steroids (although there is now some doubt over the efficacy of steroids in malignancy) and rehydration if time permits. It is hypocalcaemia which causes tetany, and this may happen if hypercalcaemia is corrected too rapidly
- Eaton-Lambert syndrome and susceptibility to neuromuscular blockade

CONDUCT OF ANAESTHESIA

This is the author's personal way of recording a general anaesthetic, and the way I teach new trainees to think and record their thoughts. As ever, it is intended to remind and prevent omissions.

Induction
Venous access on non-dominant arm for preference.

Airway
- *Means of control:* Tracheal tube, laryngeal mask or mask and airway
- Cords sprayed with lignocaine?
- Gas entry, confirmed in the anaesthetic room and again in theatre, by capnography as method of choice
- Pack? Put in capitals if you have placed an pharyngeal pack, to remind you to remove it at the end of the case
- Record the Cormack and Lehane view at intubation, so the next colleague attending the patient knows what to expect:
I   Glottis in sight, complete
II Glottis in sight, but only the posterior part
III Epiglottis only seen
IV Nothing seen. The benefit to a colleague reviewing your notes if you have recorded this is obvious

Maintenance of anaesthesia
- Spontaneous respiration (SR) or intermittent positive pressure ventilation (IPPV)?
- Machine type; record if circle used
- Gases: Record inspired oxygen fraction (FiO_2), fresh gas flow, and the volatile agent used
- Ventilation: Record minute ventilation (V_E), tidal volume (V_T), frequency of ventilation (f) and patient system pressure (PSP)

Guedel: Described stages of anaesthesia in gaseous induction using ether.

- *First stage*: Analgesia; to loss of consciousness
- *Second stage*: Excitement; to onset of automatic breathing
- *Third stage*: To respiratory paralysis
  - Plane 1: To cessation of eye movement
  - Plane 2: To start of intercostal paralysis
  - Plane 3: To completion of intercostal paralysis
  - Plane 4: To diaphragmatic paralysis
- *Fourth stage*: Overdose

Position
Record the patient position, taping of the eyes, and protection of pressure points such as elbows and the peroneal nerve at the knee.

Adjunctive anaesthesia
Regional: Epidural, brachial plexus or femoral, for example. Infiltration by surgeon or anaesthetist.

Other techniques
- Naso- or oro-gastric tube
- Pneumoperitoneum
- Table tilt
- Warming blanket
- Blood warmer
- Cell salvage
- Aprotinin

Monitors
These may be divided into those which monitor the condition of the patient, and those which monitor the equipment. One device, the capnograph, monitors both.

Patient	Equipment
Non-invasive blood pressure	Patient system pressure
ECG	Disconnection
SpO_2	O_2 failure
P_ECO_2	Gas analysis

(table continued)

Patient	Equipment
Peripheral nerve stimulator (PNS)	
Spirometry	
Temperature	
Central venous pressure	
Invasive blood pressure	
Pulmonary artery catheter	

Blood loss

From swabs and from suction.

Fluids administered

Ideally these should be timed entries, so that you can demonstrate that you responded to a drop in blood pressure, for example. The record of fluid administered must also appear on the patient's drug chart, or it may otherwise not be included in the fluid balance for the day of theatre. Bearing in mind that up to 3 litres may be administered during the course of a long, but routine, laparotomy, this volume is significant. Fluid overload is a frequent cause of admission to the intensive care unit.

Reversal

Admit to doxapram if you used it.

Postoperative instructions

Oxygen: Flow rate and duration required. Hypoxia occurs at night, and up to the third postoperative night.

Analgesia: Intramuscular opiate, patient controlled analgesia (PCA), or epidural, by infusion or top-up. Regular NSAID.

Fluids to be administered, venous access, and how long the access should be maintained. Overnight for tonsillectomy with adenoidectomy, for example.

Observations: See Postoperative Management section at the end of this chapter.

CONDUCT OF ANAESTHESIA

Machine checklist

Oxygen analyser
Calibrate to room air, and to 100% oxygen.

Gas supplies
- Disconnect pipelines and turn off cylinders
- Open all rotameters
- Turn on each O_2 cylinder and operate rotameter; set at 5 L/min
  Observe:
  - Analyser reads 100%
- Repeat for N_2O. Leave O_2 on 5 L/min
- Turn off O_2 cylinder and void system via flush valve
  Observe:
  - O_2 gauge fall
  - Audible alarm
  - Prevention of hypoxic mixture
- Connect O_2 pipeline
  Observe:
  - O_2 flow restored
  - Audible alarm silenced
- Perform 'Tug test'
  Observe:
  - 400 kPa indicated on gauge
- Repeat 6 and 7 for N_2O
- Turn off all rotameters, operate O_2 flush:
  Observe:
  - No drop in pipeline pressure
  - 100% on O_2 analyser

Vaporisers
- Secure position on backbar, free dial movement
- Flow is in correct direction
- Vaporiser full, with the correct agent, filling port closed
- If pressure relief valve (PRV) fitted, set O_2 to 6 L/min, occlude common gas outlet (CGO)
  Observe:
  - No leak
  - Dip in bobbin

- Repeat with vaporiser turned on. Unseated vaporisers are a major cause of awareness

Breathing system
- Correct configuration, no leaks, and no obstructions
- 'Push and twist' all conical fittings
- Expiratory valve opens and closes
- Bain attachment; perform occlusion test, observe bobbin drop; use oxygen flush, observe the venturi effect collapse the bag. The vulnerable point is the connection of the fresh gas flow to the inner tube. This can be confirmed visually as well
- Circle; confirm function of unidirectional valves

Ventilator
- Make it work
- Occlude patient port; observe-PRV function
- Confirm that disconnect warning alarm works
- Ensure that alternative means of ventilation is available

Suction
This is what candidates forget in the exam, apparently.

Spare laryngoscopes and tracheal tubes
Drugs drawn up
- Suxamethonium
- Atropine
- Ephedrine, whenever a regional block is used

Adapted from: Checklist for Anaesthetic Apparatus. 2. 1997. London, Association of Anaesthetists of Great Britain and Ireland.

Failed rapid sequence intubation drill

You must have an immediate action drill for this eventuality. It was first described by Tunstall in connection with failed obstetric intubation, and has been modified many times since. It is also appropriate for other situations where the airway is at risk of soiling with gastric contents. Oxygenation is paramount.

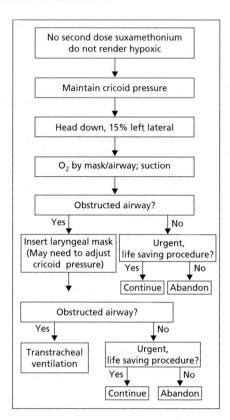

Equipment

Cylinders and gas supplies

The supply for machines in most operating theatres in the developed world is by pipeline, with cylinders as back-up. The gases are delivered at 4 bar (420 kPa, 60 psi). Oxygen comes from a vacuum insulated evaporator (VIE) at −183°C and nitrous oxide from a manifold of cylinders. After heat exchanging and pressure reduction, they enter the theatre at terminal outlets, where a Schraeder probe leads to a gas-specific hose, which in turn connects to a non-interchangeable screw thread (NIST) at the anaesthetic machine. There are either one or two pressure regulators (also called pressure reducing valves) within the machine (the number depends on the manufacturer) after which there is a pressure relief valve which operates at 800 kPa (8 bar, 120 psi) in order to protect the machine from damage. On the back bar, where the vaporisers are situated, there is a pressure relief valve which operates at 42 kPa (6 psi), which protects the patient.

There is also an oxygen failure device, which diverts the remaining gas through an audible alarm before opening the system to room air.

Cylinders for anaesthetic gases are made of molybdenum steel. Some may be fitted with a Wood's metal fusible plug in the valve block which melts at low temperature, with the intention of avoiding explosion if the cylinder is exposed to fire or other high temperature. One in every 100 is tested to destruction, and every one is tested to 10% over the working pressure every three years. The tare is the weight of the cylinder empty. Knowledge of the tare allows a full cylinder to be distinguished from an empty one.

Markings
- *Oxygen*: Black with white shoulders, sizes C-J, plus AF
- *Nitrous oxide*: Blue with blue shoulders, sizes C-G
- *Entonox*: Blue with blue and white shoulders, sizes D, F and G
- *Air*: Grey with black and white shoulders, sizes E-J
- *Carbon dioxide*: Grey with grey shoulders, sizes C, E and F
- *Cyclopropane*: Orange with orange shoulders, size B only
- *Helium*: Dark orange, sizes D and F

Sizes
- *Size B:* Tare 1.6 kg, volume 180 l, cyclopropane only
- *Size C:* Tare 2 kg, volume 170 l O_2, 450 l N_2O
- *Size D:* Tare 3.4 kg, volume 340 l O_2, 900 l N_2O, 500 l Entonox
- *Size E:* Tare 5.4 kg, volume 680 l O_2, 1,800 l N_2O
- *Size F:* Tare 14.5 kg, volume 1,360 l O_2, 3,600 l N_2O, 2,000 l Entonox
- *Size AF:* Tare 9.9 kg, volume 1,360 l O_2 only

- *Size G:* Tare 34.5 kg, volume 3,400 l O_2, 9,000 l N_2O, 5,000 l Entonox
- *Size J:* Tare 68.9 kg, volume 6,800 l O_2, 6,400 l air

Pin index
- Oxygen 2–5
- Nitrous oxide 3–5
- Cyclopropane 3–6
- Entonox 7
- Air 1–5

Physical characteristics of gases
A vapour is a substance in a gaseous state at a temperature and pressure close to those at which it would liquefy. The critical temperature is the temperature above which a vapour cannot be kept in the gaseous state by the effect of pressure alone. This does not mean that the substance, if kept in a cylinder above the critical temperature, will explode; what it means is that the contents of that cylinder will be in the gaseous phase. It would otherwise be unsafe to store nitrous oxide in the tropics. The critical pressure is the pressure required to liquefy a gas at its critical temperature.

Gas	Critical temperature (°C)	Critical pressure (bar)	Cylinder pressure (bar)
CO_2	31	72.85	50
N_2O	36.5	72.6	44
O_2	−118.4	50.14	134.7

Gauges
- The French gauge is the circumference in millimetres × 3
- The wire gauge is roughly the number of wires of that size which will pass through a 1 inch ring

Volatile agent consumption
This may be calculated from

$$(\text{Flow} \times \text{concentration})_{STP} \times \frac{MW}{22.4 \times SG}$$

STP = Standard temperature and pressure.

MW = Molecular weight of the volatile and
SG = Specific gravity of the volatile.

Flowmeters

These are commonly known as rotameters, although this is a trade term. Each is individually calibrated and lined with a very thin film of gold to prevent static making the bobbin adhere to the side and a spurious reading result. They are therefore the most expensive component of an anaesthetic machine.

Part of the flowmeter	Cross section	Type of flow	Important gas characteristic
Bottom	Tubular	Laminar	Viscosity dependant
Top	Orificial	Turbulent	Density dependant

Classification of vaporisers and breathing systems

Conway classification

This is the classic way of describing a breathing system.

- *Open:* No exclusion of ambient air, no confinement of exhaled gases
- *Semi-open:* Partial exclusion of ambient air, partial confinement of exhaled gases; an example is the Schimmelbusch mask
- *Semi-closed:* Fully bounded system, with provision for gas overflow; examples include the Bain and Magill attachments
- *Closed:* A fully bounded circuit, no overflow of exhaled gases; the only example is a circle with the expiratory valve screwed down and a minimum fresh gas flow

Dorsch and Dorsch

This is a way of describing a vaporiser in an exam.

- *Method for regulating concentration*: Variable bypass or measured flow
- *Method of vaporisation*: Flowover or bubble-through

- *Location*: In or out of circle. A plenum system is one where the pressure within is greater than the pressure without. Most contemporary vaporisers are plenum vaporisers, and cannot be used as drawover vaporisers as the resistance to flow is too great
- *Temperature compensation*: None, supplied heat or bimetallic strip
- *Specificity*: For different vapours

Mapleson classification

This is the classical way of describing a breathing attachment. Few of them are circular, so describing them as circuits is inappropriate.

In all cases, the arrow indicates the fresh gas entry and the bar indicates the adjustable pressure relief valve. Mapleson was a professor of the Physics of Anaesthesia.

- *Mapleson A:* The Magill attachment is the classical example of this

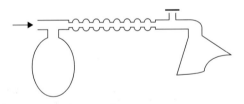

- *Mapleson B:*

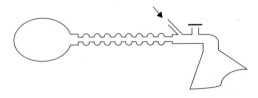

- *Mapleson C:* The Waters to-and-fro, used for transferring patients and for physiotherapy on the intensive care unit

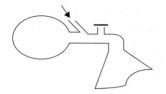

- *Mapleson D:* The Bain attachment is functionally a Mapleson D arrangement

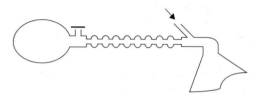

- *Mapleson E:* Ayres' t-piece

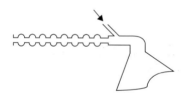

Mapleson did not describe F, but the expression is much used to describe Jackson-Rees' modification of Ayres' t-piece:

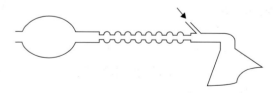

Gas and ventilation
Fresh gas flows
- For spontaneous respiration:
  - *Bain (Mapleson D):* 2–3 × minute ventilation
  - *Magill (Mapleson A):* Alveolar ventilation

- For controlled ventilation:
  - *Bain:* 70 ml/kg/min to keep $PaCO_2$ 5.3 kPa
  - *Ayres' t-piece:* 2–3 × minute ventilation, and in any case more than 4 l/min. The volume of the limb must exceed tidal volume or dilution of fresh gas with room air occurs
- For circles:
  - Low flow is defined as less than 3 l/min. To perform this safely, most would advocate the use of agent and carbon dioxide monitoring

Ventilation values

In the awake resting state these may be calculated as follows:

Body weight (kg)	Minute volume, V_E (ml)	Tidal volume, V_T (ml)
2	480	14–16
3	600	17–24
7	1,000	50–60
10	1,680	80

Thereafter: $V_T = 8$ ml/kg;
$V_E = 4,000$ ml for 30 kgBW
   $= 5,600$ ml for 70 kgBW

Pressure conversions

Different machines use different units of pressure. They may also use different units from those used in physiology. Converting between them all is a problem, but a few calculations may help.

$$1\,atm = 1\,bar = 1,000\,millibars$$
$$= 101\,kPa = 101,000\,N/m^2$$
$$\approx 15\,psi$$
$$= 760\,mmHg = 760\,Torr.$$
$$1\,kPa \approx 10\,cmH_2O = 100\,mmH_2O$$

So; $100\,kPa = 15\,psi$
       $1\,kPa \approx 0.15\,psi$
       $1\,psi \approx 6.66\,kPa$

And; $100\,kPa = 760\,mmHg$
$1\,kPa = 7.6\,mmHg$
$10\,mmHg = 1.32\,kPa$

Regarding the sitting patient: $1\,cmH_2O = 0.76\,mmHg$. Thus the perfusion pressure of the head falls by $0.76\,mmHg$ from the recorded pressure at chest level for every $1\,cm$ that the head is above the level of the chest. This is of relevance in surgery in the sitting position, especially if hypotension has been deliberately used.

Harvard minimum monitoring standards

These were implemented to reduce malpractice premiums but have become accepted as the basis of good anaesthetic practice since then.

- Presence of anaesthetist throughout procedure and until patient fully recovered
- ECG
- Blood pressure and heart rate measured and recorded every 5 min
- Observation of ventilation: Movement of the bag, or monitoring breath sounds, or end-tidal CO_2
- Observation of the circulation: Palpation of pulse, or SpO_2
- Disconnection alarm
- Measurement of FiO_2

The ability to record patient temperature was added as a footnote.

Eichorn JH, Cooper JB, Cullen DJ, Maier WR, Philip JH, Seeman RG: Standards for patient monitoring during anaesthesia at Harvard Medical School. *JAMA* 1986; 256: 1017–20.

Capnography

Capnography is possibly the single most useful monitor in general anaesthetic practice.

Definitions:

- *A Capnograph* is a device which records and displays the CO_2 concentration
- *A Capnogram* is a graphical plot of CO_2 as a function of time
- *A Capnometer* is an instrument for measuring the numerical concentration of CO_2. Thus, all capnographs are capnometers, but a capnometer need not display a capnogram
- *Realtime:* A capnogram waveform displayed at 12.5 mm/sec, demonstrating fine detail and sudden changes in morphology
- *Trend:* A capnogram waveform displayed at 25 mm/min, demonstrating gradual changes over time
- *Delay time:* The sum of the transit time and the rise time
- *Transit time:* The time taken for a sample to be delivered from the point of interest to the analyser
- *Rise time:* The time taken by the capnographic cell to register from 10% to 90% of a step change after the sample has entered the measuring chamber. The latter is also known as the response time, and is important as it must be less than the time taken for one breath
- *Mainstream:* Where the analysing cell is interposed in the breathing system. These do not cause turbulent flow in the breathing system nor do they extract gas from it (both of importance in paediatric anaesthesia) and they have a short delay time, but they are vulnerable to being dropped and damaged. They are also heavy and difficult to support when using a mask. They heat up
- *Sidestream:* Where a continuous sample is drawn at the rate of 150 ml/min from the breathing system to be analysed within the machine. This is the more common arrangement, but the gas needs to be scavenged, or returned to the system if a circle is in use. Condensation forms and a water-trap is needed
- *Infrared analysis:* This uses absorption of infrared light
- *Mass spectrometry:* This uses deviation of ions in a magnetic field
- *Raman scattering:* The shift in photon frequency following interaction with a molecule

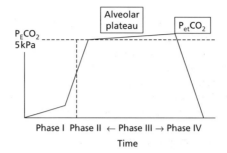

Patterns associated with particular disorders

- *Malignant hyperpyrexia:* High peak PCO_2
- *Chronic airways disease:* Slow upstroke, wide $P(a-ET)CO_2$ gradient
- *Defective valves in a circle system:* Raised baseline with oscillations
- *CO_2 rebreathing:* Raised baseline, with oscillations in phase IV
- *Circulatory arrest:* Progressive diminution in amplitude
- *Oesophageal intubation:* Even with carbonated drink in stomach, less than 6 deflections will be seen. Thereafter, the tube cannot be in the trachea if no CO_2 is detected, unless circulatory arrest has occurred
- *Airway obstruction:* Slow ascent phase II
- *Recovery from neuromuscular blockade during positive pressure ventilation:* Clefts are seen during phase III

Nitrous oxide absorption

- *Initially:* 400 ml/min
- *After 1 h:* 75 ml/min
- *After 3 h:* 20 ml/min

Absorption is governed by a process of two time constants, of 25 and 500 min respectively.

Oximetry

This may be pulse oximetry (*in vivo*) or bench oximetry (haemolysed sample, *in vitro;* co-oximetry). The advantage of bench oximetry is that it can differentiate between different species of haemoglobin (e.g. COHb, MetHb)

Pulse oximetry

Light is transmitted across a digit or extremity from an LED to a photodiode, at two wavelengths, 660 and 940 nm. Reduced Hb absorbs better at 660 nm and oxygenated Hb at 940 nm. They are the same at the isobestic point (803 nm). The non-pulsatile component of the signal (venous blood, unless a venous pulse is present, e.g. tricuspid incompetence) is subtracted by a microprocessor, leaving the arterial component to be measured.

It is most accurate above 90% saturation, and much less accurate below 70%. These devices are calibrated against healthy volunteers, which makes calibration to values below 70% ethically unacceptable. Problems leading to inaccuracies include:

- Diathermy
- Motion
- Vasoconstriction
- Venous engorgement and pulsation
- Bile and dyes
- Abnormal Hb (especially COHb, which gives a spuriously high reading)
- Ambient light

Neuromuscular monitoring

- *Nerve stimulator:* Delivers 50 mA for 0.2–1.0 msec; requires 50–300 V
- *Twitch-tetanus-twitch:* This distinguishes the *type* of block; four patterns are observed
  1. *Normal:* symmetrical twitches followed by sustained tetanic contraction; no post-tetanic facilitation (PTF)
  2. *Total block:* No response
  3. *Partial depolarising block:* Weak but symmetrical twitches, sustained tetanic contraction, no PTF
  4. *Partial non-depolarising block:* Weak twitches, fade on tetanic stimulus, PTF

- *Train of four:* This distinguishes the *degree* of block.
  - Count 1,2,3   75% block
  - Count 1,2   80% block
  - Count 1   90% block
  - Count 0   100% block
- *Post-tetanic twitch count:* This determines the *reversibility* of a block; the device delivers 50 Hz for 5 sec, then 1 Hz, counting detectable twitches. Reversal is possible if count is greater than 10
- *Double burst:* This uses 3 pairs of 50 Hz pulses separated by 0.75 sec. It assesses *recovery* from block, displaying the T1:T4 ratio

Endobronchial tubes

Indications for use
- Absolute indications (these are usually anaesthetic reasons):
  - Rupture or fistula
  - Massive haemorrhage
  - Bronchoplastic procedures: One-lung transplant
- Relative indications (usually surgical):
  - Lung resection
  - Oesophageal surgery

Identification of types
The smallest available are 26 FG. Observe and describe: Lumens, cuffs, pilot balloons, oropharyngeal and bronchial curves, orifices (especially if in a cuff), and suction orifices.

Confirmation of placement
Fibreoptic examination is the definitive method.

The key is to *isolate* the upper, operative lung and to *ventilate* the dependant, lower lung.
- Inflate tracheal cuff: Hear BS over both lungfields
- Inflate bronchial cuff, deflate tracheal cuff: Hear sounds only on bronchially-intubated side
- Then ventilate each side separately
- Repeat after patient movement

The surgeon will invite you to 'let the lung down'. To do this, clamp the tracheal lumen (red marking) and remove the bung from the top of its tube; the bronchially-intubated (blue marking) tube will now ventilate the dependant lung, and the upper lung will be isolated and should deflate. If there is a leak around the bronchial cuff, however, the upper lung may reinflate.

The considerable shunt which is imposed by the deflation of one lung must be monitored by oximetry. It may be alleviated by:

- Surgical ligation of the pulmonary artery on the upper side: This closes the shunt
- Periodic reinflation of the operative, upper lung, with the surgeon's cooperation
- Insufflation of the upper lung with 100% oxygen

Use of pressure-volume and flow-volume loops displayed on a monitor during surgery will identify the secondary displacement of an endobronchial tube from its original position, because the appearance of the loops will alter with time.

The laryngeal mask airway (LMA)

Inventor A I J Brain
Number of prototypes >60
First commercial production 1988

Size	Maximum inflation volume (ml)	
6	50	Large adult male
5	40	Adult male
4	30	Adult female
3	20	Small adult female/teenager
2½	14	20–30 kg child
2	10	10–20 kg child
1½	7	5–10 kg
1	4	up to 5 kg

Insert by following the path of deglutition.

Laryngeal mask insertion can be facilitated by attention to detail. Lubricate the back of the mask. Inflate with a small amount of air. Insert by pushing the tip of the mask along the curve of the hard and soft palates. This allows gentle pharyngeal entry and avoids folding back the epiglottis. Occasionally a gloved finger may be used to flip the tip of the mask as it touches the posterior pharynx. Inflate the mask gently and slowly.

A correctly positioned LMA under light anaesthesia may result in an obstructed airway. This can often be improved by deepening anaesthesia.

Avoid LMA movement during light anaesthesia as this may precipitate laryngospasm especially in children and infants. At the end of anaesthesia leave the patient undisturbed until airway protection reflexes have returned. At this time the patient will often swallow retained saliva and be able to open their mouth for airway removal.

In children, the LMA should be removed in the same way as a tracheal tube.

Position on the table

The structures at risk, from head to toe, are:
- The supraorbital nerve in the prone position
- The elevation of orbital venous pressure in the prone position
- The upper airway when the stomach is above the airway
- The shoulder joint abducted in the prone position
- The brachial plexus compressed in the lateral position
- The brachial plexus at median sternotomy
- The ulnar nerve at the elbow in flexion
- Left ventricular output from venous air embolism where veins are open above the right atrium, in neurosurgery and when the uterus is open
- The lungs from diaphragmatic elevation due to anaesthesia, and abdominal compression in the prone position
- The distal venous system from thrombosis formation in lithotomy
- The common peroneal nerve from lithotomy poles

Regional anaesthesia

Local anaesthetic agents
There are two groups of local anaesthetics; esters and amides. Ester local anaesthetics such as procaine, cocaine and

- Maternal symptoms such as severe headache and epigastric pain (which arises from stretching the liver capsule)

Foetal
- Distress
- Severe IUGR
- Reversed umbilical artery diastolic flow

PET protocol
Once a mother is included onto the protocol there is a commitment to delivery of the foetus within 24 h and often within 12 h.

Diagnostic inclusion criteria
Either 1 or 2 or 3.
1. Hypertension greater than 140/90, plus $\geq 2+$ proteinuria and at least one of: Platelets below 100,000, urate >0.45 or AST over 25, oliguria <500 ml in 24 h, clonus more than 3 beats
2. Severe hypertension greater than 170/110
3. Eclampsia

Fluid
- Hartmanns solution 85 ml/h (this needs reducing if other infusions are running)
- If urine output <0.5 ml/kg/h for 4 h a fluid bolus can be given. Check no evidence of pulmonary oedema and that oxygen saturation is satisfactory on air. The mother may also feel thirsty. A bolus of 250 ml of colloid can be given over 15 min which can be repeated once
- If oliguria persists, institute central venous pressure (CVP) monitoring. PA catheter insertion may occasionally be necessary as RA and LA pressures do not correlate well in PET

Antihypertensives
- If mean arterial pressure (MAP) is ≥ 125 mmHg for more than 45 min then antihypertensive treatment should be started. Preload with 500 ml colloid over 20 min

- Labetalol 10 mg i.v. which can be repeated every 5 min. An infusion can also be used starting at 6–10 mg/h. Titrate rate to keep MAP <125 mmHg.
- Alternatively, hydralazine 5 mg by slow i.v. injection, which can be repeated at 15 min intervals. Side effects include tachycardia and headaches
- Nifedipine 10 mg sublingually can be given in refractory cases

Anticonvulsants
- Magnesium sulphate is now the anticonvulsant of choice both for treatment and prevention of fits
- Loading dose of 4 g
- Maintenance 1 g/h
- If further fits occur, a further 2 g i.v. bolus can be given
- Plasma levels are not routinely measured at these infusion rates unless there is renal impairment. However, reflexes should be routinely monitored to check these are still present. At high plasma concentrations, magnesium will reduce conscious level and muscle tone, and can even cause respiratory embarrassment. Magnesium should not be used for myaesthenics or for mothers taking calcium channel blockers

Antacid prophylaxis
- Ranitidine 50 mg slowly i.v. 6 hourly

Anaesthesia for LSCS
- Incremental top up of epidural
- If no epidural *in situ*, a CSE using a low dose spinal followed by incremental epidural top ups provides smooth BP control. Give 1 ml 0.5% hyperbaric bupivacaine, 25 mcg fentanyl and 0.5 ml saline intrathecally. Follow with epidural tops ups of 0.5% bupivacaine 3–5 ml
- Post operative analgesia can be provided by an epidural infusion of 0.1% bupivacaine and 2 mcg/ml fentanyl at 10–20 ml/h
- If a syntocinon infusion is required, this can be given as a small volume via a syringe driver to minimise fluid load

Peribulbar block

- *Position:* Supine
- *Landmarks:* Medial canthus, at caruncle; apply 1% amethocaine to conjunctiva
- *Needle:* 25 G, 25 mm short bevel, perpendicular to skin, parallel to septum
- *Endpoint:* Just short of end of needle
- *Injection:* 8 ml 2% lidocaine with hyalase 500 u

Interscalene block

- *Position:* Supine, arm by side, invite to sniff or to lift head slightly off pillow to identify interscalene groove
- *Landmarks:* Cricoid cartilage, level of C6; interscalene groove. This block lends itself to being performed with a nerve stimulator
- *Needle:* Insulated 25 G
- *Endpoint:* Eliciting twitches in arm
- *Injection:* 20 ml 0.5% bupivacaine

Axillary block

- *Position:* Supine, hand abducted, elbow flexed, hand pronated
- *Landmarks:* Pulsation of axillary artery within sheath
- *Needle:* Insulated 25 G
- *Endpoint:* Eliciting twitching in arm. Some recommend transfixion of the artery
- *Injection:* 20 ml 0.5% bupivacaine

Stellate ganglion block

- *Position:* Supine
- *Landmarks:* Transverse process of C6: Chassaignac's tubercle
- *Needle:* Short level, 25 G
- *Endpoint:* Bone; withdraw fractionally
- *Injection:* 5 ml 2% lidocaine

Three-in-one block

- *Position:* Supine
- *Landmarks:* Immediately lateral to the pulsation of the femoral artery
- *Needle:* 22 G insulated needle, 5 cm
- *Endpoint:* Quadriceps twitch at 0.3–0.4 mA
- *Injection:* 20 ml 0.5% bupivacaine

Postoperative management

Recovery instructions

When handing over to the recovery staff, the following are the five essential items of information:

1. Patient's name
2. Nature of operation and duration of anaesthetic
3. Whether intubated or not
4. Concurrent illness of relevance to the immediate postoperative period (e.g. measure glucose and restart dextrose and insulin infusion)
5. Analgesia provided so far, and plans for postoperative period

The instructions to recovery staff may be considered under the following headings:

- Timing and frequency of observations required
- Oxygen therapy to be given, and duration
- Duration of monitoring of oxyhaemoglobin saturation
- Respiratory rate which is acceptable
- Heart rate and rhythm which is acceptable
- Blood pressure which is acceptable
- Conscious level required
- Adequacy of pain relief: Be ready to accept that a patient is in pain and do not withhold analgesia where it is needed

It is a Royal College recommendation that there should be an acute pain service whereby all patients with either an epidural or PCA are seen every day by an anaesthetist, who may also be contacted at any time for advice. No patient with a PCA or an epidural may receive night sedation or opiate medication by any other route. Some authorities insist on High-Dependency Unit (HDU) care for patients who have received spinal opiates. It is usual to prescribe a non-steroidal anti-inflammatory drug in conjunction with these techniques. Analgesia will otherwise be administered by the nursing staff in accordance with the anaesthetist's instructions. If it is necessary to prescribe additional analgesia, consider why it has become necessary – has something changed or gone wrong – bleeding into a joint, perforation of a viscus, etc., before writing up a stronger preparation

Never prescribe a NSAID in renal impairment, dehydration, aspirin-sensitive asthma, peptic ulceration, or risk of bleeding

Never sedate a chronic bronchitic, especially of the CO_2 retaining type; use opiates with caution in these people

- Dermatomal level of regional block to be maintained if a regional technique has been used for postoperative pain relief
- I.V. access and fluids: A diuretic must *under no circumstances* be administered without knowledge of the fluid balance and clinical state of hydration, and preferably with the knowledge of the central venous pressure. The correct treatment of oliguria in the first instance is a fluid challenge of 3.5 ml/kg body weight of colloid. This may need to be repeated depending on response; See 'Fluid and replacement' in the Physiology section
- Postoperative drugs
- Operation site review
- Other; CVP, urine output, temperature

Post operative acute pain management guidelines

To be effectively treated pain should be anticipated rather than responded to. All recommendations made are for regular prescriptions not PRN. All prescriptions should be reviewed daily. Not for use in pregnancy.

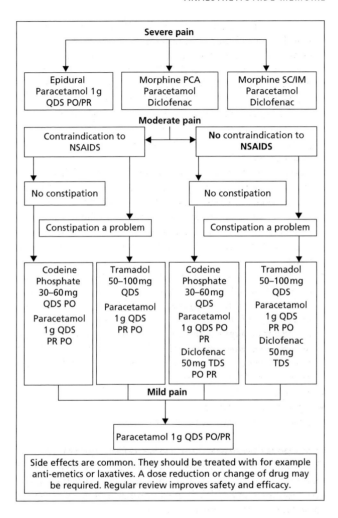

NSAIDS

Consider any contraindications due to:
- History of GI perforation/ulcer/bleed
- Allergy/renal impairment/hypovolaemia
- NSAID/aspirin sensitive asthma
- Bleeding risk.

Opioids

Consider reducing the dose or increasing the time between doses in:
- Renal/hepatic impairment. Elderly/debilitated.

Guidelines for the treatment of nausea and vomiting in adults after surgery

Consider prescribing **cyclizine** four doses 25–50 mg on the regular side of the drug chart for patients having a PCA. If a patient has past history of PONV or it is anticipated that the PCA may be used for a longer period more doses may be required.

Indications for the first line use of **Ondansetron** are:
- Past history of extrapyramidal reaction to cyclizine.
- Specific operations including adenotonsillectomy in children, squint correction and middle ear surgery.

Dexamethasone dose may be repeated once during the next 24 h. Not for use in pregnancy. Contraindicated in sepsis or infection. Caution with exogenous steroids and diabetes mellitus.

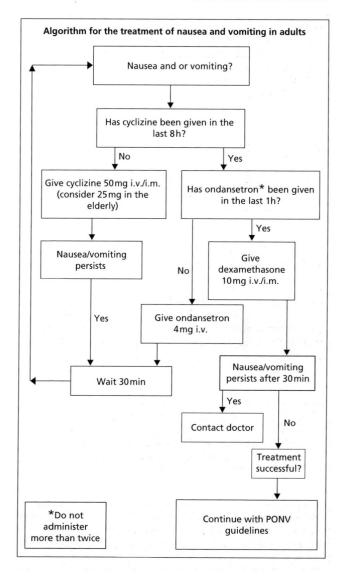

Algorithm for the treatment of nausea and vomiting in adults

Nausea and or vomiting?

Has cyclizine been given in the last 8h?

No → Give cyclizine 50 mg i.v./i.m. (consider 25 mg in the elderly)

Yes → Has ondansetron* been given in the last 1h?

Give cyclizine → Nausea/vomiting persists

Has ondansetron* been given in the last 1h? → Yes → Give dexamethasone 10 mg i.v./i.m.

No → Give ondansetron 4 mg i.v.

Nausea/vomiting persists — Yes → Wait 30 min

Give dexamethasone / Give ondansetron → Nausea/vomiting persists after 30 min

Nausea/vomiting persists after 30 min → Yes → Contact doctor

No → Treatment successful?

Treatment successful? → Continue with PONV guidelines

*Do not administer more than twice

CONDUCT OF ANAESTHESIA

Algorithm for intermittent subcutaneous opioid injection

Adults only

Notes

Not for use in pregnancy

Every patient should have a i.v. cannula *in situ* for emergency use

Weight	Morphine
Elderly/debilitated or <44 kg	5 mg
45–65 kg	7.5 mg
>66 kg	10 mg

The subcutaneous cannula is the dedicated injection port for opioids only. Label it.

Respiratory depression: Draw up to 0.4 mg (1 ml) of naloxone + 3 ml of normal saline and give in 1 ml increments (i.v.) until resp rate >12, and sedation score less than 2.

Termination

If the pain score is 1–4 and 4–6 h has elapsed since the last i.m. injection, consider oral analgesia.

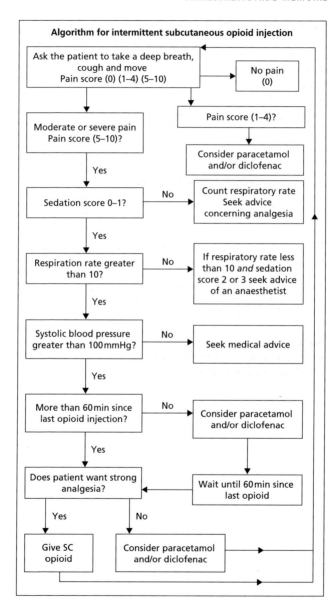

Algorithm for intermittent subcutaneous opioid injection

Ask the patient to take a deep breath, cough and move
Pain score (0) (1–4) (5–10)

No pain (0)

Pain score (1–4)?

Consider paracetamol and/or diclofenac

Moderate or severe pain
Pain score (5–10)?

Yes

Sedation score 0–1? — No → Count respiratory rate
Seek advice concerning analgesia

Yes

Respiration rate greater than 10? — No → If respiratory rate less than 10 *and* sedation score 2 or 3 seek advice of an anaesthetist

Yes

Systolic blood pressure greater than 100mmHg? — No → Seek medical advice

Yes

More than 60min since last opioid injection? — No → Consider paracetamol and/or diclofenac

Yes

Does patient want strong analgesia? ← Wait until 60min since last opioid

Yes — Give SC opioid

No — Consider paracetamol and/or diclofenac

Epidural management on a surgical ward

Inadequate analgesia consider
- Infusion rate too low
- Epidural catheter insertion site
  - Lumbar for pelvic surgery
  - Thoracic for abdominal or chest surgery

One sided block
- Top up
- Position patient pain side down
- Pull back catheter (optimum 3–4 cm in the epidural space)

Pump failure
- Battery
- Line detached (usually at the filter)
- Line kinked
- Line blocked with blood or at filter junction

Catheter not in the epidural space

Cardiovascular
Hypotension
- Hypovolaemia or vasodilatation. Fluid challenge with colloid 250 ml, repeat if required. Consider using ephedrine
- Bradycardia can be due to sympathetic block at T1-T4, in which case treat with atropine and turn infusion off

Others
- Excessive sedation, turn pump off treat with naloxone or resuscitation if required
- Itching treat with naloxone

Effective doses usually are:
- Bupivacaine   8–15 mg/h
- Ropivacaine   8–15 mg/h
- Fentanyl   0.5–1.0 mcg/kg/h

The co-administration of paracetamol where suitable will often lower a pain score.

Remember to ask ward staff to perform observations according to local protocol after a top up or significant change in infusion rate.

Both systemic local anaesthetic overdose and total spinal anaesthetic are rare. They are medical emergencies requiring management of airway breathing and circulation and a call for senior help.

Paediatric analgesic doses

Drug	Dose	Route	Interval	Preparation
Para-cetamol	*Oral*: Loading dose 20 mg/kg then 10–15 mg/kg. Maximum oral dose 80 mg/kg/day up to 1 g 6 h (60 mg/kg/day under 3 months).	PO	4–6 h	*Syrup:* 120 mg/ 5 ml or 250 mg/ 5 ml
	Rectal: Loading dose 20–40 mg/kg (20 mg/kg for neonates) then 20 mg/kg. Maximum rectal dose 100 mg/kg/day up to 1 g 6 h (80 mg/kg/day day under 3 months).	PR		*Supps:* 60, 120, 240, 500 mg
Ibuprofen	5 mg/kg/dose. Maximum 4 doses per day. Not recommended if under 7 kg. Caution in asthmatics.	PO	6 h	*Syrup:* 100 mg/ 5 ml
Diclofenac	1 mg/kg/dose. Maximum 3 mg/kg/day. Not under 1 y of age. Caution in asthma.	PO/PR	6–8 h	*Supps:* 12.5, 25, 50, 100 mg
Codeine Phosphate	1 mg/kg/dose. Maximum 6 mg/kg/day. Not recommended under 1 y. Never give	PO/PR i.m. in theatre	4–6 h	*Syrup:* 15 mg/5 ml or 25 mg 5 ml *Inj:* 60 mg/ml

(table continued)

Drug	Dose	Route	Interval	Preparation
	intravenously – causes hypotension.			
Morphine Sulphate	Oral: 200–400 μg/kg over 1 y. Children under 1 y with consultant advice.	PO	6 h	Syrup: 10 mg/5 ml OR 30 mg/5 ml
	Intravenous: 50 μg/kg boluses up to 100–200 μg/kg intravenously.	i.v. bolus		
	PCA: see separate protocol, basically 1 mg/kg (up to 50 mg) of morphine in 50 ml 0.9% saline with 1 ml bolus (20 μg/kg) and 10 min lockout.			

Entonox® is very useful to consider for short procedures in children over approximately five years of age. Cylinders are available from A&E. Should be administered under medical supervision.

Anti-emetic doses

Drug	Dose	Route	Interval	Preparation
Ondansetron	100–200 μg/kg. Maximum 4 mg/dose.	PO/i.v.	8 h	Syrup: 4 mg/5 ml Inj: 4 mg/2 ml
Cyclizine	1 mg/kg to maximum of 50 mg.	PO/i.v.	8 h	Inj: 50 mg/ml
Dexamethasone phosphate	250 μg/kg to maximum 8 mg.	i.v.	Single dose	Inj: 8 mg/2 ml

Diazepam

Can be a useful adjunct if muscle spasms are a problem. Twice daily oral dosages:

Age (years)	Tranquillising (mg)	Spasms (mg)
1–4	0.5	2.5
5–12	1–1.5	5
≥13	2	10

Midazolam

For pre-med 500 µg/kg *orally* to a maximum dose of 15 mg for pre-med 30–45 min pre-op *only* if required. The intravenous preparation is given orally in this situation.

Intramuscular injections should be avoided if possible on the paediatric ward.

Analgesic *combinations* should be prescribed whenever possible; *regular* analgesics should always be considered.

Appropriate consent should be obtained before rectal administration.

These doses are guidelines only and should be prescribed with reference to the British National Formulary and paediatric formularies (e.g. 'Medicines for Children') which are available on the paediatric ward.

Day case unit discharge criteria

- Adequate ventilation established
- Patient is awake and lucid
- Observed stability of blood pressure and heart rate and rhythm
- Swallow and cough reflexes restored
- Walking without fainting
- No nausea or vomiting
- Patient has passed urine
- Patient has taken fluids
- Operation site reviewed
- Postoperative instructions given, verbally and in writing, and understood by patient and carer

- Postoperative therapy provided
- GP letter sent
- GP phoned if indicated
- Follow-up arrangements made
- Supervision confirmed

Day case discharge instructions

- Instructions about observations given to carer
- Patient to be accompanied by an adult of 'suitably robust proportions', responsible for care for next 24 h
- Analgesia and postoperative instructions provided in written form with contact phone numbers in case of difficulty
- Warning given, pre- and postoperatively, in verbal and written form, against driving, operating machinery, cooking, childminding, and against the ingestion of alcohol or sedative drugs other than those prescribed, for a minimum of 24 h

Postoperative pyrexia

This can be due to four common causes, which may be neatly summarised as follows:

- 2 days: *Wind*: Chest infection
- 4 days: *Water*: Urinary tract infection
- 6 days: *Wound*: Abscess
- 8 days: *Walk*: Deep vein thrombosis

PHYSIOLOGY

Haemodynamic variables

Pressures: Normal values

Variable	Formula	Normal value
Cardiac output	$CO = SV \times HR$	5 L/min
Cardiac index	$CI = \dfrac{CO}{BSA}$	3.2 L/min/m²
Stroke volume	$SV = \dfrac{CO}{HR} \times 1,000$	80 ml
Stroke index	$SI = \dfrac{SV}{BSA}$	50 ml/m²
Systemic vascular resistance	$SVR = \dfrac{MAP - CVP}{CO} \times 80$	1,000–1,200 dyne-sec/cm²
Pulmonary vascular resistance	$PVR = \dfrac{PAP - LAP}{CO} \times 80$	60–120 dyne-sec/cm²
Ejection fraction	$EF = \dfrac{ESV - EDV}{EDV}$	>0.6, or ×100 expressed as a percentage

Ejection fraction is a really useful index as it describes the performance of the left ventricle at rest, and can only be one of three things; Good, >70%; moderately impaired, 40–70%; or severely impaired, <40%.

Pressures

Right atrial pressure	1–7 mmHg (2–10 cmH₂0)
RV systolic	15–25 mmHg
RV diastolic	0–8 mmHg
PA systolic	15–25 mmHg
PA diastolic	8–15 mmHg
Pulmonary artery pressure (PAP)	10–20 mmHg
Pulmonary capillary wedge pressure (PCWP)	6–15 mmHg

The arterial pressure signal

At least four things can be learnt from the arterial pressure signal.

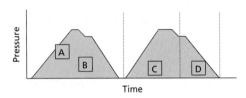

A: Rate of pressure increase is proportional to myocardial contractility.
B: Area under the curve of pulse pressure is proportional to stroke volume.
C: Systolic pressure × time is proportional to myocardial work and O_2 consumption.
D: Diastolic pressure × time is proportional to myocardial perfusion.

Arterio-venous oxygen difference and mixed venous oxygen

Taking simultaneous arterial and mixed venous (the latter from the tip of a pulmonary artery catheter) samples allows for derivation of the arterio-venous oxygen difference. The Fick equation permits calculation of VO_2, oxygen consumption.

Fick:

$$\dot{Q} = \frac{\dot{V}O_2}{CaO_2 - C\bar{v}O_2}$$

Reverse Fick:

$$\dot{V}O_2 = CO \times \left(CaO_2 - C\bar{v}O_2\right) \times 10$$

For CaO_2 and $C\bar{v}O_2$:

$$O_2 \text{ content} = (1.39 \times Hb \times Sat/100) + 0.02 \, PO_2$$

The VO_2 can then be assessed in the light of the cardiac output at that time. Shoemaker (*Intens Care Med* 1987; 13: 230–43) suggests that the critically ill patient requires a VO_2 30% greater than normal (N = 100–180 ml/min/m²). Many people now regard this, and the other Shoemaker goals, as more of a physiological test than a set of achievable targets.

Mixed venous oxygen

Mixed venous oxygen saturation is the percentage of mixed venous blood which is oxygenated, and may be measured photometrically at the tip of a PA catheter.

$S\bar{v}O_2$ is decreased with:
- Anaemia
- Low cardiac output
- Arterial oxygen desaturation
- Increased oxygen consumption

$S\bar{v}O_2$ is increased with:
- Sepsis with peripheral shunting
- Cyanide toxicity
- Hypothermia
- A wedged PA catheter

Venous pulse

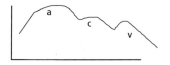

a = Atrial systole. A cannon wave is a massive a-wave seen in complete heart block.
c = Bulging of tricuspid valve in isovolumetric ventricular systole. Increased in tricuspid incompetence.
v = Atrial filling.

PHYSIOLOGY

Lung volumes, capacities and loops

A capacity consists of two or more volumes. Figures shown are for an adult.

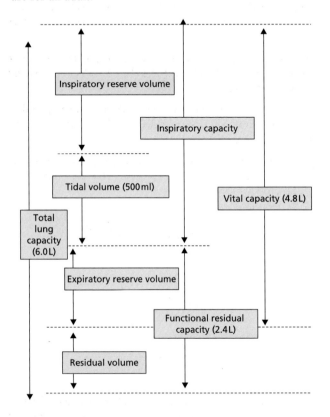

Closing capacity = Closing volume + Residual volume

This rises with age and represents the volume of the lungs at which small airways start to close. Functional residual capacity (FRC) is reduced by 20% in anaesthesia due to diaphragmatic shift, decreased ribcage dimensions and positive pressure ventilation. If FRC falls below CC, areas will be perfused but not ventilated. This explains at least part of the V/Q mismatch seen in anaesthesia and is one reason for the use of inspired fractions of oxygen of at least 0.30.

Maximum breathing capacity = Maximum frequency × vital capacity (VC), sampled over 15 sec; normal value is greater than 60 l/min; less than 25 l/min represents severe respiratory incapacity.

Forced vital capacity (FVC) reduction implies restrictive disease; normal is 60 ml/kg. If less than 15 ml/kg, the patient is unable to cough.

The ratio of the forced expiratory volume in one second to the forced vital capacity is the (FEV_1/FVC ratio) reduction implies obstructive disease.

Pressure- and flow-volume loops

Pressure-volume loops

These are about:

$$Compliance = \frac{volume}{pressure}$$

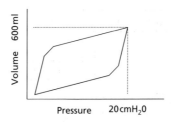

This is an example of hysteresis. In addition to quantification of disease (restrictive airways disease), it is used to represent graphically the efficiency or inefficiency of ventilation – for example, when more pressure produces no more volume. It may also demonstrate the secondary displacement of an endo-bronchial tube.

Compliance × Resistance = The time constant, of a particular lung unit. Differing time constants within a lung represent disease and will cause pendelluft, with inefficiency of gas movement. Compliance may decrease at high frequency in this case, and dynamic, rather than static, compliance becomes a more meaningful measurement.

Flow-volume loops

These are about:

$$Resistance = \frac{pressure}{flow}$$

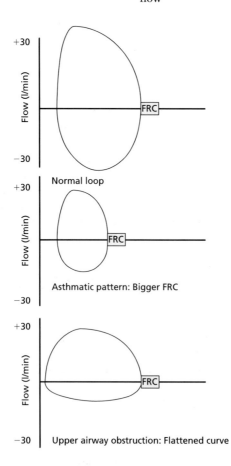

Normal loop

Asthmatic pattern: Bigger FRC

Upper airway obstruction: Flattened curve

Single breath nitrogen test

This is a modification of Fowler's method: The patient takes a slow expiration after a single breath of 100% O_2, and the nitrogen concentration in the expiration is measured. A perpendicular drawn through phase II locates $V_{D,anat}$. The slope of phase III (the alveolar plateau) defines evenness of ventilation distribution. The start of phase IV defines closing capacity.

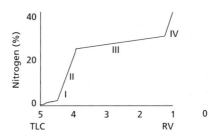

The oxyhaemoglobin dissociation curve (ODC)

This relates the percentage of haemoglobin in the blood which has oxygen bound to it, to the local partial pressure of oxygen. It is best drawn through a series of known points; I have chosen the P_{50}, the P_{90} and venous blood.

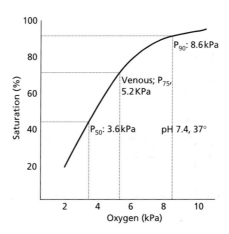

- Hb rapidly takes on O_2 when in the pulmonary capillary
- Hb retains O_2 until it reaches regions of relative hypoxia
- Hb is 50% saturated (P_{50}) at a partial pressure of 3.6 kPa, and 90% saturated (P_{90}) at 8.6 kPa
- The Bohr Effect is shifting of the ODC to the right, which means that binding will be inhibited and unloading of O_2 facilitated. This is caused by: $\uparrow CO_2$, $\uparrow$ Temperature, $\uparrow [H^+]$ and $\uparrow$ 2,3 Diphospho glycerate (DPG)

Physics and equations

These are the commonly-used equations, listed here for reference. A very few notes of explanation are given to explain the relevance of an equation to anaesthetic practice.

Ideal gas equation:

$$PV = RT$$

Where P = pressure; V = volume; T = temperature, and R = constant. At the same temperature, P and V are inversely related; increasing pressure will reduce volume.

Dead space:

$$V_{D,Phys} = V_{D,Anat} + V_{D,Alv}$$

Total dead space ($V_{D,Phys}$) is made up of alveolar dead space (non-ventilated alveoli) and anatomical dead space (conducting airways). Alveolar dead space increases in disease while anatomical dead space increases with age.

Bohr equation:

$$V_D/V_T = \frac{P_A CO_2 - P_E CO_2}{P_A CO_2}$$

The Bohr equation assumes no CO_2 in inspired gas. The normal physiological (total) dead space, as a proportion of tidal volume $(V_D/V_T) = 0.3$.

To measure $V_{D,Anat}$: Fowler's method; corresponds to vertical line through phase II of the single breath nitrogen washout. Normal = 150 ml.

Alveolar ventilation equation:

$$\dot{V}_A = \frac{\dot{V}CO_2}{P_ACO_2} \times K$$

Where $K = 0.863$, if V_A is body temperature, ambient pressure, and saturated with water vapour (BTPS), and VCO_2 is standard (0°C) temperature and pressure (760 mmHg) and dry (STPD). Essentially, alveolar ventilation is proportional to CO_2 production and inversely proportional to alveolar CO_2.

This is not the same as what follows (although it is a common mistake to confuse the two):

Alveolar gas equation:

$$P_AO_2 \propto P_IO_2 - \frac{P_ACO_2}{R}$$

The alveolar partial pressure of oxygen is dependant on the inspired fraction and on the amount of CO_2 which is effectively, displacing the oxygen. This explains the advantage of pre-oxygenation, and explains why desaturation occurs rapidly after apnoea as the CO_2 accumulates in the alveoli unless pre-oxygenation has been used. It also relates to altitude, and explains the mild hyperventilation seen at altitude – reduction in CO_2 allows more space for oxygen. The equation as written above assumes no CO_2 in inspired gas.

Venous admixture: This is venous blood entering the systemic arterial circulation. Venous admixture is due to frank shunt + The effects of low V/Q. Note that while V/Q affects O_2 and CO_2, shunt only really affects oxygenation.

Shunt equation:

$$\frac{\dot{Q}_s}{\dot{Q}_t} = \frac{Cc'O_2 - C_aO_2}{Cc'O_2 - C\bar{v}O_2}$$

Normal = 5 ml/100 ml.

Diffusing capacity:

The amount of gas transferred across a membrane is proportional to: Area, difference in partial pressures, constant and 1/thickness.

Diffusing capacity may be measured by the single breath carbon monoxide (CO) technique, where the disappearance of a single breath of CO is measured over a 10 sec breath hold. Helium dilution is used to measure total lung volume at the same time.

$$D_L = \frac{\dot{V}CO}{P_ACO}$$

(Normal 25 ml/min/mmHg)

Oxygen flux = Cardiac output × Oxygen content.

Oxygen content = (1.39 × Hb × Sat/100) + 0.02 PO_2

Henderson-Hasselbalch:

$$pH = pKa + \frac{\log(HCO_3^-)}{0.03 PCO_2}$$

This is used to calculate blood pH, which falls (blood becomes more acid) if the bicarbonate falls or the CO_2 rises.

Laplace's law:

$$P = \frac{2T}{r}$$

Where P is the pressure in a bubble, T is the surface tension and r is the radius. A small bubble (or alveolus) will collapse into a large one because it will have a larger pressure within it, due to the action of T in the walls of the alveolus. This does not happen, of course, because of the action of surfactant, which reduces the surface tension .

Pouseille's law:

$$Q = \frac{P\pi r^4}{8\eta l}$$

Where Q is the flow through a tube, P is the pressure difference between the ends, η is the viscosity of the fluid and l is the length of the tube. Laminar flow applies. The point is that flow through a tube, vessel or cannula is determined by the driving pressure, the viscosity and the length in a simple manner but is governed by the radius of the tube to the fourth power. So, doubling the radius of a cannula increases flow 16 times.

Fanning equation:

$$Q = \frac{P\pi^2 r^5}{fr}$$

This is analogous to Pouseille's law but describes turbulent, not laminar, flow.

Reynolds number:

$$Re = \frac{2rvd}{\eta}$$

This describes the possibility of turbulent flow, where r is radius, v is velocity and d is density, with η is viscosity as before. If the number exceeds 2,000, turbulent flow is likely.

The Bernoulli effect is that gas passes faster through a constriction, gaining kinetic energy, but losing potential energy and so dropping pressure. If used to entrain a second gas, this is the Venturi effect. The Coanda effect is that a substance flowing in a tube is attracted to the walls. This is the basis of some ventilators.

Other respiratory gas curves

The shunt diagram
This is used to demonstrate the effect of different degrees of shunt on arterial oxygenation, in the presence of increased inspired fraction of oxygen (FiO_2). Essentially, if no shunt is present, PaO_2 will increase linearly with FiO_2. However if a large shunt is present, increasing the FiO_2 will not improve oxygenation.

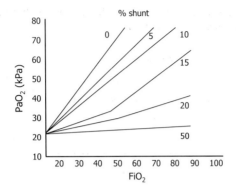

The O_2 – CO_2 diagram

Alveolar CO_2 and alveolar O_2 cannot alter independently one of the other; they are related. This diagram is used to display all the possible combinations of alveolar CO_2 and O_2 that can exist. A is the arterial combination, with a PO_2 of about 13 kPa and PCO_2 5.2 kPa. I is the inspired combination, with atmospheric oxygen and no carbon dioxide. V is the mixed venous combination. These points are joined by a line, movement along which is governed by alterations in V/Q, as shown.

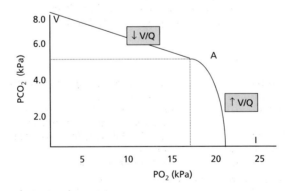

The CO_2 response curve

This relates ventilation V, to arterial CO_2. This is one of the few relationships which is truly linear, and is displaced to the right (requiring a higher CO_2 for the same ventilation) by general anaesthesia and sedation.

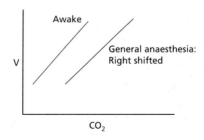

Fluids and replacement

To calculate normal blood volume
- *Adult:* 7% Body Weight (Body water = 42 L in 70 kg man) or, 70 ml/kg
- *Child:* 80 ml/kg
- *Neonate:* 90 ml/kg

Daily water requirement

0–10 kg body weight	5 ml/kg/h
10–20 kg body weight	add 2 ml/kg/h
>20 kg body weight	add 1 ml/kg/h

Nutritional requirement

Potassium	1.5 mmol/kg/day (1 g = 13.5 mmol)
Sodium	1.0 mmol/kg/day
Energy	in kCal = water requirement in ml
	25–35 non-protein kCal/kg/day
Nitrogen	0.2–0.4 g N_2/kg/day (monitor urea)
Magnesium	1 mmol/g N_2
Phosphorus	0.5–0.75 mmol/kg/day

Water soluble vitamins
Trace elements: Zn^+ 100 μmol, Cu^{++} 20 pmol, Mn 5 μmol, Se 0.4 μmol.
Essential fatty acids
Maximal rate of glucose infusion = 6.0 mg/kg/min

Intraoperative fluid requirement

Add $1 + 2 + 3 + 4$ = Total requirement

1. *Initial volume:* 1.5 ml/kg/h for duration of period of starvation
2. *Maintenance:* 1.5 ml/kg/hr for duration of operation
3. *Insensitive loss:* e.g. opened peritoneum 1 L
4. *Blood loss:* Transfuse if loss is $>20\%$ blood volume. However this needs to be interpreted in the light of the starting haemoglobin. It has been traditional for patients to have a haemoglobin >10 g/dl for elective surgery. This is due to concerns for myocardial supply. The myocardium extracts 12 ml/dl of oxygen from every 100 ml of blood delivered to the coronary circulation. The CaO_2 of blood with a Hb of 10 g/dl is 14.5 ml/dl. This comfortably exceeds the maximum extraction from the myocardial supply

Burns fluids

There are a number of ways of calculating the requirement for burns fluids. One of the best known is the Muir and Barclay formula, which covers colloid, crystalloid and blood.

Colloid: (Body weight $\times$ % body surface burn (BSB))/2 = ml to be transfused per block; blocks occupy 4, 4, 4, 6, 6, 12 h post injury.

Crystalloid: metabolic requirement as 5% dextrose 1.5 $\times$ BW $\times$ ml/h.

Blood: 50 ml/1% BSB.

Static plasma deficit: This allows calculation of how the resuscitation of a burns victim is proceeding. Take calculated blood volume (BV):

$$\text{Deficit (ml)} = BV - \frac{(BV \times \text{Normal Hct})}{\text{observed Hct}}$$

Chemistry and correction

The tendency to tetany

This is proportional to

$$\frac{[HCO_3^-] \times [HPO_4^-]}{[Ca^{++}] \times [Mg^{++}] \times [H^+]}$$

Such that the risk is enhanced by high bicarbonate and a low hydrogen ion concentration (in other words, by alkalosis) and by a low calcium ion concentration.

Anion gap

This is a measure of the presence of acid moieties. It is calculated:

$$([Na^+] + [K^+]) - ([Cl^-] + [HCO_3^-])$$

Normal = 10–15 mmol/l

The anion gap is increased by:	The anion gap is decreased by:
Increased serum lactate – but lactate can be directly measured now, so the anion gap has become a less frequently used measurement	Hypoalbuminaemia
Ketoacidosis	Increased plasma cations
Increased foreign anions, salicylates for example	
Low Ca^{++}, Mg^{++}, K^+	

Calculation of osmolarity

$$= 2[Na^+ + K^+] + [Urea] + [Glucose]$$

Normal = 285–295 mOsm/l

Direct measurement by depression of freezing point indicates osmolality. Calculation indicates osmolarity. In reality, there is little difference between osmolarity and osmolality other than when there is extreme hyperlipidaemia or hyperproteinaemia. Comparison of plasma and urine must be done in terms of osmolality of both, in other words, by direct measurement.

Correction of acidosis

Base deficit (ecf) × kg body weight/3, given as ml of 8.4% Bicarbonate (1 ml = 1 mmol).

Usually, half of this is given and a repeat measurement taken. Chemical correction of acidosis is only used if the acidosis is extreme and if respiratory correction has been unsuccessful.

Blood coagulation pathways

Primary haemostasis depends solely on platelet function. The coagulation proteins form Fibrin which stabilises the platelet clot.

The intrinsic pathway is so-called because all components circulate in plasma:

$\Downarrow$ = action; $\rightarrow$ = conformational change

Intrinsic: Platelets   *Extrinsic:* Cell damage
      $\Downarrow$ Tissue thromboplastin III
XII $\rightarrow$ XIIa $\Downarrow$
  XI $\rightarrow$ XIa   VII $\rightarrow$ VIIa
    IX $\rightarrow$ IXa $\Downarrow$
   VIII $\rightarrow$ VIIIa
          $\Downarrow$ Ca$^+$ $\Downarrow$
     X $\rightarrow\rightarrow\rightarrow\rightarrow\rightarrow\rightarrow\rightarrow$ Xa
              Ca$^+$ $\Downarrow$
   Prothrombin II $\rightarrow\rightarrow\rightarrow$ IIa   XIII
                $\Downarrow$ $\Downarrow$
        Fibrinogen I $\rightarrow$ Fibrin $\rightarrow$ Polymer

Tests of coagulation

Platelet count	>150,000/mm^3
Fibrinogen	>150 mg/100 ml
Platelet function	Bleeding time <10 min
Intrinsic (heparin)	KCCT (APPT) <38 sec
Extrinsic (warfarin)	PT <16 sec

This may also be given as the International Normalised Ratio (INR) to a control using a standard thromboplastin. The ratio required depends on the condition, e.g. 2 for prophylaxis against emboli in atrial fibrillation, and 3 where a prosthetic valve is to be protected. The KCCT can also be quoted as a ratio.

Warfarin

This is a vitamin K antagonist causing false synthesis of γ-carboxyglutamic acid residues at factors as below:

Factor	VII	IX	X	II
Half-life	2 h	17 h	40 h	60 h

Dose of warfarin: 10 mg od, until adequate INR is achieved, then maintenance with 1/4 total initial dose. Reversal is possible with Vitamin K 10 mg and fresh frozen plasma if urgent.

Heparin

This is an antithrombin III cofactor; 100 u = 1 mg. Initial dose 5,000 u, then 1,000 u/h. Heparin 4 mg/kg is used during coronary artery bypass grafting. Reversal is by protamine 1 mg/100 u heparin. Protamine must be given with caution and slowly as a reversal dose of protamine for 4 mg/kg of heparin will consist of up to 25 ml of the standard 1% solution. Protamine causes a drop in systemic vascular resistance and an increase in pulmonary vascular resistance, and these effects are enhanced in the presence of high inspired oxygen fractions.

Low molecular weight heparin (LMWH)

Fractionated heparin (LMWH), is a once daily dose, and is more popular in orthopaedic practice. Need factor X assay to monitor effect. Less reversible with protamine.

Thrombolysis

```
Vascular endothelium → Prostacyclin = Platelet inhibitor
Plasminogen
    ↓     ⇐ Tissue plasminogen activator (tPa)
    ↓     ⇐ Kallikrein }
    ↓     ⇐ XIIa        } both from intrinsic pathway
Plasmin ⇒ Cleavage of fibrin and fibrinogen
                    ↓                ↓
                Fibrin degradation products
```

Tests:

Fibrin degradation products (FDP); normal <10 mg/ml.

D-dimer: FDP portion released only in fibrinolysis; normal <500 ng/ml.

PHARMACOLOGY AND STATISTICS

Pharmacokinetics is the study of what the body does to a drug, in contrast to pharmacodynamics, which is the study of what a drug does to the body. Kinetics allow for the prediction of action of drugs in normality and in altered states of metabolism.

Single compartment models
Where the drug is resident in, and eliminated from a single space.

First-order kinetics
Rate of elimination is proportional to amount of drug present, X.

$$\frac{dx}{dt} = -kX$$

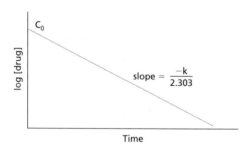

Volume of distribution

$$V_d = \frac{X_0}{C_0}$$

where X_0 is drug quantity at time 0, and C_0 is concentration at time 0.

Half-Life

$$t_{\frac{1}{2}} = \frac{0.693V_d}{Cl}$$

Independent of X_0, but dependent on volume of distribution, V_d and clearance, Cl.

Two-compartment model

This is where the drug in question is resident in, and moves between, two spaces in the body and is eliminated from one or the other. Thiopentone is an example of this, where the rapid offset of action is due to redistribution from the plasma (the first compartment) to lipid-rich tissue, the second compartment.

α = Rate constant of distribution phase
β = Rate constant of elimination phase
A and B = Intercepts

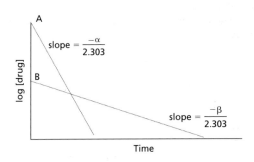

$$Cl = \frac{X_0}{AUC}$$

where AUC = Area under the curve.

The major implications are:
- $t_{\frac{1}{2}}$ independent of dose
- AUC is proportional to dose
- Steady state achieved after $t_{\frac{1}{2}} \times 4$ regardless of dose
- Loading dose = Desired plasma level $\times V_d$
- Infusion rate = [steady state] $\times Cl$
- A drug will accumulate if the dose interval, T < 1.4 $\times t_{\frac{1}{2}}$

Non-linear pharmacokinetics

Some drugs behave as if rate-limited by the capacity of their elimination system. These include alcohol, phenytoin and salicylates. The Michaelis-Menton equation describes saturable enzyme kinetics but can be applied to the mathematical modelling of non-linear kinetics:

$$\frac{dC}{dt} = \frac{V_m C}{K_m + C}$$

where V_m = Apparent max rate of process, K_m = [drug] at half max rate and C = [drug].

The implications of this are:
- If C is far below K_m, first-order kinetics apply
- If C is far above K_m, the decline in concentration proceeds at a fixed rate; this is zero-order kinetics
- The time required to eliminate 50% of dose increases with increased dose: No constant $t_{1/2}$
- AUC is proportional to square of the dose; small increase in dose can cause huge increase in amount of drug in body, once elimination process is saturated
- More than one drug may use the same route of elimination in which case competition occurs

Pharmacodynamics

This is the study of what the *drug* does to the *body*. In contrast to pharmacokinetics, this is very difficult to model mathematically as the mechanism of action of drugs is complex, systems may become saturated, and plasma values of a drug may bear little resemblance to the concentration at the site of action; psychotropic drugs are examples. A drug may have complicated effects which outlast the presence of the agent itself; steroids are an example of this. Finally, some agents do observe a close relationship between amount present and observed effect; these are mostly receptor based in their action and include remifentanil at the μ receptor, inotropes on α and β receptors, and nitroprusside in its action on smooth muscle.

PHARMACOLOGY AND STATISTICS

The log dose-response curve is the typical diagram used to describe pharmacodynamic relationships. The use of logarithms allows for curved relationships to become linear, interactions to be more easily spotted and for easier calculation of effective doses.

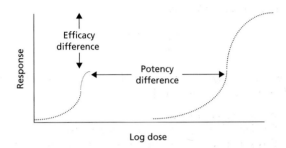

For example, fentanyl is more potent than alfentanil, so the log dose-response curves will be the same shape (that is, both reaching 100% response) but they will be separated on the x-axis. Dihydrocodeine is not as efficacious as fentanyl, so the log dose-response curves for these two drugs will not be the same shape, the curve for dihydrocodeine never reaching the same height on the y-axis as fentanyl.

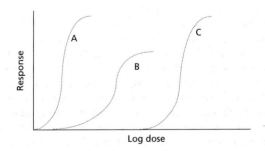

A: Drug with high affinity and high intrinsic activity: True agonist: Fentanyl.
B: Drug with high affinity but less intrinsic activity: Partial agonist; never reaches 100% response: Buprenorphine.

C: Agonist in presence of antagonist; Agonist will reach 100% response even in the presence of the antagonist, as long as the dose of agonist is great enough: Fentanyl and naloxone.

The ideals

The ideal induction agent
Physical
- Water-soluble
- Stable in solution
- No adsorption onto plastic
- Cheap to synthesise
- Compatible with other drugs

Pharmacokinetic
- Sleep in one arm-brain circulation time
- Short and predictable duration of action
- Not cumulative
- Inactivation by metabolism to inactive metabolites

Pharmacodynamic
- No pain on injection
- No cardiovascular or respiratory effects
- Analgesic
- No histamine release
- No increase in muscle tone or excitatory movements
- No interactions
- No effects on the gravid uterus
- Safe if extravasated or given intra-arterially

Total intravenous anaesthesia (TIVA)

This is the technique of using an induction agent both for induction of anaesthesia and as a continuous infusion to maintain anaesthesia. It avoids the use of volatile agents. This may be useful in avoiding nausea, vomiting, enhancement of neuromuscular blockade, atmospheric pollution and the risk of Malignant Hyperpyrexia. There is a risk of awareness if disconnection occurs; also, Minimum Infusion Rate (which is analogous to minimum alveolar concentration (MAC)) is poorly defined for most agents.

These are some examples:
- *Propofol* 1% 50 ml, mixed with *Alfentanil* 1.5 mg; 1.0 mg/kg propofol for induction, followed by 10 mg/kg/h, then 8 mg/kg/h then 6 mg/kg/h. This may be used for spontaneously breathing or paralysed and ventilated patients
- *Propofol* 1% 50 ml mixed with *Remifentanil* 2 mg, induction midazolam 3 mg sleep dose propofol, followed by 15–25 ml/h when combined with an epidural. Epidural analgesia needs to be established before waking. Unlicensed use.

Administration of TIVA

This is by syringe driver although the earliest examples used simple drip sets.

CLAN is closed loop anaesthesia and involves use of the auditory evoked response to adjust the amount of TIVA administered.

The ideal inhalational agent

Physical
- Stable in light, heat, metal, sodalime
- No preservatives
- Long shelf life
- Not flammable or explosive in air, N_2O or oxygen
- Non-irritant
- Atmospherically friendly
- Cheap to synthesise

Pharmacokinetic
- High oil:gas coefficient, so low MAC
- Low blood:gas coefficient, so fast effects
- Not metabolised

Pharmacodynamic
- Non-toxic, even in chronic, low dose
- No cardiovascular or respiratory effects
- Analgesic
- Readily reversible central nervous system (CNS) effects
- Not epileptogenic
- No interactions
- No effects on the gravid uterus

Characteristics of volatile anaesthetic agents

	MAC	BP	SVP	B:G	O:G	MW
Halothane	0.7	50	33%	2.3	224	197
Enflurane	1.7	56	24%	1.8	98.5	184
Isoflurane	1.17	49	33%	1.4	99	184
Sevoflurane	1.9	55	24%	0.6	53	200
Desflurane	6.0	23	88%	0.4	20	168

MAC: The amount of the agent delivered in oxygen at room temperature at sea level which will keep 50% of unpremedicated experimental animals still at skin incision.

It is reduced by:
- Age (10% per decade)
- Premedication
- Opioids
- Hypovolaemia
- Reduced temperature
- Other drugs: For example, clonidine, dexmedetomidine
- Disease: Hypothyroidism

BP: Boiling point, in °C

SVP: The pressure exerted by the vapour phase above the liquid phase at equilibrium, in other words when as many molecules are leaving the liquid as returning. This depends on the agent and its temperature and is independent of atmospheric pressure. It defines the calibration of the vaporiser.

B:G: Blood:Gas partition coefficient: The less soluble the agent, the more rapid the onset and offset of action.

O:G: Oil:Gas partition coefficient: This bears a linear inverse relationship to MAC and is therefore an indicator of potency.

MW: Molecular weight, in Daltons.

Calculation of infusion rates

1% = 10 mg in 1 ml;
1:10,000 = 1 g in 10,000 ml

1 ml = 15 normal drops = 60 microdrops
∴ 1 ml/h = 1 microdrop/min

1 L over 12 h = 83 ml/h = 20 drops per min
1 L over 8 h = 125 ml/h = 30 drops per min
1 L over 6 h = 166 ml/h = 40 drops per min
1 L over 4 h = 250 ml/h = 60 drops per min

To calculate infusion rates:
3 mg of drug into 50 ml
(1 ml/h = 1 mcg/min)

By body weight
Body weight in kg × 3 mg of drug into 50 ml
(1 ml/h = 1 mcg/kg/min)

Common infusions: adults

Drug	Presentation	Dose
Epinephrine	1 mg ampoule (1:1,000)	0.1–1.0 mcg/kg/min
Alfentanil	5 mg ampoule	0.5–1.0 mcg/kg/min
Aminophylline	250 mg ampoule	0.2–0.9 mg/kg/h
Amiodarone	150 mg ampoule	5 mg/kg; 5 mcg/kg/min
Dopamine	200 mg ampoule	1.0–15 mcg/kg/min
Dopexamine	50 mg ampoule	0.5–6.0 mcg/kg/min
Dobutamine	250 mg ampoule	2–10 mcg/kg/min
Fentanyl	0.5 mg ampoule	0.02–0.05 mcg/kg/min
GTN	50 mg ampoule	5–20 mcg/min
Lidocaine	1 gr ampoule	100 mg loading dose, 2–4 mg/min
Magnesium sulphate	5 g ampoule	1–2 g loading dose, 2–2.5 g/h
Nitroprusside	50 mg ampoule	0.5–10 mcg/kg/min
Norepinephrine	2 or 4 mg ampoule	4.0–12 mcg/min

Relaxants

Neuromuscular blockade is usually maintained by the use of non-depolarising agents, very few practitioners still favour the intermittent suxamethonium technique. Non-depolarisers can be given by intermittent bolus or by infusion.

Vecuronium 10 mg in 5 ml of buffered freeze-dried bromide as powder for reconstitution. Contains mannitol.	Dose (mcg/kg)	Dose (mg for a 70 kg patient)	Volume of dose for 70 kg (ml)
Intubation	100	7	3.5
Maintenance (Bolus)	50	3.5	1.7
Maintenance (Infusion)/h	80	5.5	2.5
Atracurium 50 mg in 5 ml yellow coloured solution of the besylate; stored at 2–8°C	Dose (mcg/kg)	Dose (mg for a 70 kg patient)	Volume of dose for 70 kg (ml)
Intubation	600	40	4
Maintenance (Bolus)	200	15	1.5
Maintenance (Infusion)/h	600	40	4
Rocuronium 50 mg in 5 ml clear solution of the bromide.	Dose (mcg/kg)	Dose (mg for a 70 kg patient)	Volume of dose for 70 kg (ml)
Intubation	600	40	4
Maintenance (Bolus)	150	10	1
Maintenance (Infusion)/h	600	40	4

Inotropes

Drug	Property	Dose
Dopamine	D > β > α	2.5 mcg/kg/min
Dobutamine	β1 > β2 > α	5–20 mcg/kg/min
Epinephrine	α, β1, β2	0.1–1.0 mcg/kg/min
Norepinephrine	α > β1	4–12 mcg/kg/min
Dopexamine	β2 > β1 > D	0.5–6 mcg/kg/min
Ephedrine	α > β1 > β2	3–6 mg increments

(table continued)

Drug	Property	Dose
Metaraminol	α	1–2 mg increments
Phenylephrine	α	100–500 mcg bolus
Salbutamol	β2 > β1	3–20 mcg/min

Note: Adrenaline = epinephrine
Noradrenaline = norepinephrine

Antiarrhythmics

Antiarrhythmics control the rhythm of the cardiac contraction usually by reducing the excitability of the conducting system or of the myocardium.

The cardiac action potential (AP)

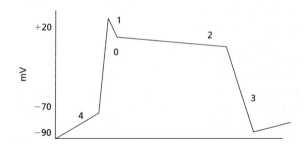

0 = Fast depolarisation, Na^+ inwards
1 = Early incomplete repolarisation
2 = Plateau, slow Ca^{++} inwards, prolonging AP
3 = Rapid repolarisation, K^+ outwards
4 = Electrical diastole, refractory period.

Vaughan-Williams classification

Ia $\downarrow Na^+$ entry in phase 0; $\uparrow$repolarisation; disopyramide
Ib $\downarrow Na^+$ entry in phase 0; $\downarrow$repolarisation; lignocaine, mexilitine
Ic $\downarrow Na^+$ entry in phase 0; flecainide
II β-blockade; propranolol, metoprolol

III ↑repolarisation; bretylium, amiodarone
IV Ca^{++} blockade; verapamil, nifedipine.

Recommendations for specific arrhythmias

- *Ventricular arrhythmias:* Lidocaine 100 mg then 2–4 mg/min, or mexilitine
- *Atrial fibrillation without compromise:* Digoxin 1 mg divided in 24 h, then 125–150 mcg/day; or DC shock after anticoagulation and stopping digoxin
- *Atrial fibrillation with compromise:* DC Shock
- *Fast atrial fibrillation of recent onset:* Flecainide 2 mg/kg then 1.5 mg/kg in one hour then 100–250 mcg/kg/h
- *Wolff-Parkinson-White syndrome:* Amiodarone 5 mg/kg slow bolus then 200 mg/day
- *Supraventricular tachycardia of recent onset:* Adenosine 3 mg, doubling until effect seen
- *Supraventricular tachycardia:* Verapamil 5–10 mg slow bolus
- *Torsades des pointes:* Magnesium 4 g bolus then infusion 1 g/h, aim for 2–3.5 mmol/l

Paediatric dosages and calculations

Drugs

Premedicants

Atropine	20 mcg/kg
Glycopyrrolate	40 mcg/kg
Trimeprazine	2 mg/kg
Diazepam	0.1–0.2 mg/kg
Promethazine	0.5–1.0 mg/kg
Midazolam	0.5 mg/kg oral

Antiemetics

Ondansetron	100–200 mcg/kg

At the neuromuscular junction

Atracurium	0.5 mg/kg
Neostigmine	50 mcg/kg
Bupivacaine	Caudal to L4: 0.5 ml/kg of 0.25%, up to 2 mg/kg
	Caudal to T6: 1 ml/kg of 0.25%, up to 2 mg/kg
	Lumbar: 0.75 ml/kg of 0.25%, up to 2 mg/kg

(table continued)

Resuscitation	
Adrenaline	0.1 ml/kg of 1:10,000
Bicarbonate	1 mmol/kg
Lignocaine	1 mg/kg
DC shock	1–2 J/kg

Dehydration

Appears at loss of 5% of circulating volume = 50 ml/kg

Obvious at loss of 10% of circulating volume = 100 ml/kg

Manifest at loss of 15% of circulating volume = 150 ml/kg

Daily fluid requirement

0–10 kg body weight	100 ml/kg/day
10–20 kg body weight	add 50 ml/kg/day
>20 kg body weight	add 20 ml/kg/day
4 ml/kg/h in theatre	

Blood replacement

Blood volume 90 ml/kg (neonate), 80 ml/kg (child).

Transfuse 10 ml blood/kg body weight for every g/dl required.

Note that paediatric cardiac index is twice that of an adult = 4.8–6.0 L/min/m^2, and that oxygen consumption, VO_2 is also twice the adult = 6.8 ml/kg/min.

Ventilation

The Newton valve

- Set times and pressures estimate volumes
- Inspiratory time 1.0 sec
- Expiratory time 1.5 sec
- Peak inspiratory pressure 15 cmH$_2$O
- FiO$_2$ 0.3
- Fresh gas flow 1.0 l + (200 ml/kg) per minute

Paediatric endotracheal tube sizes

Neonate:

- 10 cm tube, 3.0 mm internal diameter

Over three months

- Internal diameter (mm) = Age/4 + 4
- Length (cm) = 12 + Age/2

The epidural space

Depth in cm is $1 + 0.15 \times$ age (y), or $0.8 + 0.05 \times$ weight (kg).

It should be located using loss of resistance to saline to avoid the risk of venous air embolism, which can be catastrophic. A test dose with adrenaline will not reliably detect venous placement.

Misuse of drugs regulations

Schedules refer to the regulations governing the use of drugs, from the Misuse of Drugs Regulations 1985.

Classes refer to the harmfulness of the drugs and the penalties for misuse, from the Misuse of Drugs Act, 1971, which replaced the Dangerous Drugs Act.

- *Schedule 1:* Includes non-medicinal drugs such as cannabis and lysergide.
- *Schedule 2:* Imposes requirements for prescribing cocaine, heroin, morphine. Full dispensing record must be kept. Drugs kept in locked container.
- *Schedule 3:* Includes barbiturates and buprenorphine; subject to special prescribing requirements, but not to safe custody requirements; nor is a register required.
- *Schedule 4:* Includes the benzodiazepines. As for *Schedule 3*, but no special prescribing requirements.
- *Schedule 5:* Includes preparations which require only retention of invoices for two years.

- *Class A:* Alfentanil, morphine, opium, heroin, methadone, pethidine, cocaine, LSD, injectable amphetamines.
- *Class B:* Oral amphetamines, cannabis, codeine.
- *Class C:* Amphetamine derivatives, and most benzodiazepines.

Cannabis is to be moved from Class B to Class C in the UK.

Statistics

Statistics is a range of techniques and procedures for describing or analysing data, and for making decisions based on data.

A population is an entire set of objects, observations or scores that have something in common, e.g. all anaesthetists.

A sample is a subset of a *population*, e.g. anaesthetists at West Suffolk Hospital (WSH).

A variable is a measured characteristic which differs between individuals, e.g. systolic blood pressure.

A parameter is a number quantifying some aspect of a *population,* e.g. mean systolic blood pressure of all anaesthetists.

Quantifying the parameters of a distribution tells you everything about it.

Considering a circle, if you know where its centre is, and what its radius is, you know everything there is to know about it. The position of its centre and its radius are its parameters. Considering a straight line, its slope and y-intercept define it uniquely, and are thus its parameters. The parameters of a normal distribution are its mean and standard deviation. The mean tells you the most frequent value; the standard deviation tells you how spread out the values are. Know these parameters, and there is nothing more to know.

All distributions have their own parameters. These depend on what things you need to know to define the distribution fully and unambiguously.

The term parameter is also used extensively by the brain dead upon their entry into middle management to try (unsuccessfully) to distract attention from their dismal lack of education.

A statistic is a number derived from a *sample* from which a *parameter* of the *population* can be estimated, e.g. mean systolic blood pressure of anaesthetists at WSH.

N.B the mean blood pressure of all anaesthetists is a parameter of the normal distribution which describes the sbp's of all anaesthetists. It is defined as the expected systolic blood pressure of an anaesthetist, and is thus theoretical and largely unknowable. This parameter is symbolised by the Greek letter μ.

One can however take a sample from that population, such as the WSH anaesthetists, measure their blood pressures, and calculate the statistic M, also called the mean, by adding them up and dividing by the total number.

This statistic M will enable you to estimate the value of the parameter μ for the whole population. The bigger the sample, the better the estimate.

Note that many named quantities have two parallel existences: they can mean a parameter which describes a distribution, or can mean a statistic which describes a sample. Parameters have Greek letters, statistics have Latin ones. Standard deviation, probability and correlation all inhabit this dual world.

In summary, if you measure the systolic blood pressures of a sample of anaesthetists, add them up, and then divide by the number in the sample, you calculate the statistic M, or arithmetic mean of the sample. This statistic enables you to estimate the parameter μ, or mean of the normal distribution which describes the population of all anaesthetists.

A normal (Gaussian) distribution is a frequency distribution where most scores are concentrated around a central figure (the mean). Above and below this figure, the number of scores falls off smoothly and continuously, resulting in a symmetrical bell shaped curve.

To good approximation, one standard deviation either side of the mean contains 66% of a normal distribution. Two s.d's contain 95% of the distribution, and 3 s.d's contain over 99%.

The normal distribution has a precise mathematical definition, worked out by Gauss. It is of interest because an inordinately large number of things in nature follow the normal distribution. There is however nothing normal about it. If you ask me, it's rather odd.

The mean of a score in a sample is its average value.

The median of a score in a sample is the value above and below which equal numbers of measurements have been made.

The mode is the most frequently observed value.

These are measures of central tendency, and are all the same if the distribution is symmetrical.

The standard deviation is a statistic calculated from a sample to reflect the degree to which the individual scores are spread out.

For each score, its difference from the mean is calculated. All these differences are squared (which gets rid of the minus signs). The squares are added up and divided by one less than the sample size, to make a sort of average called the variance. The square root of the variance is the standard deviation.

The range is the biggest minus the smallest score.

The interquartile range is the difference between the 25th and 75th percentile.

Place all the scores in order: The interquartile range is the difference between the score a quarter of the way down the list, and the score three quarters of the way down the list.

These are measures of spread or dispersion.

A sampling distribution is the frequency distribution of a statistic when repeated samples are taken.

Imagine taking repeated samples of 10 people, measuring their blood pressures, and calculating an arithmetic mean for each sample. Each time you do it, you will get a different answer, but there will be a tendency for the sample means to cluster around the true mean blood pressure μ of the whole population. The sample means are normally distributed around the population mean, even when the population itself is not normally distributed. The degree to which the sample means are spread out will depend on the dispersion of the underlying population σ and on the sample size. If you take samples of three people at a time, their means will be all over the place. If you take samples of thirty, they will all have a mean of 120 mmHg, give or take one or two.

The standard deviation of the means derived from repeated sampling is called the standard error of the mean.

Any statistic derived from sampling has its own standard error.

The standard error of the mean in a sample is given by the standard deviation of the population σ divided by the square root of the number in the sample. The standard error of the mean is therefore always less than the standard deviation of the underlying population. For big samples, it is much less.

A confidence interval is the range of values that has a specified probability of containing the parameter being estimated.

Inferential statistics are used to draw inferences about a population from work done on a sample.

Probability is the likelihood of something happening. It is expressed as a number between 0 and 1 such that a probability of 0 refers to an impossible outcome, and a probability of 1 represents an inevitable outcome.

The probability of an outcome in a population is represented by the Greek letter π. Where a probability is a statistic derived from a sample it is called p.

Which test to use?

Interval scale normally distributed data	*Ordinal* and non-normally distributed interval scale data	*Nominal* data
Two groups Unpaired t-test	Mann-Whitney U-Test	
One group Paired t-test	Wilcoxon signed-rank test	χ^2 Test
Multiple groups One-way anova Two-way anova	Kruskal-Wallace test Friedman test	

t-Test produces t value and, depending upon degrees of freedom, p is then read from a table.

$$t = \frac{\bar{d}}{SE}$$

$$\text{Variance} = \frac{\sum (x - \bar{x})^2}{n - 1}$$

$$\text{Standard deviation} = \sqrt{\frac{\sum (x - \bar{x})^2}{n - 1}}$$

$$\text{Standard error of the mean} = \frac{SD}{\sqrt{n}}$$

Research and publishing

Writing a protocol

This precedes the setting up of a trial and is an important part of the process; it will be seen by the members of the Ethics Committee of the hospital where the study will be taking place.

- *Title:* Explain project and name investigations
- *Introduction:* Need for work
- *Aim:* One sentence
- *Statement of problem:* Enlarges introduction
- *Details of method:* Exact procedure; possible problems and way around them
- *Analysis and interpretation:* Include power of study and statistical methods
- *Application of findings:* Practical benefit
- *Proposed schedule:* Start and finish, duration of each part
- *Facilities available:* Involvement of other departments, e.g. biochemistry
- *Finance*

Writing a paper

It is conventional to set out a paper as follows. Always adhere to the published guidelines of the journal to which you intend submitting the paper.

- *Abstract:* Why, how, findings, meanings
- *Key words:* From MeSH headings
- *Introduction:* What is known, what needs doing
- *Materials and methods:* What I used, what I did, to whom, how. Statistical methods used
- *Results*
- *Discussion:* Implications, are conclusions valid, agreement with others, more research needed
- *Acknowledgements*
- *References*

Vancouver criteria for authorship

This sets out what is required for an individual to be considered worthy of authorship; (a), (b) and (c) must all be met.

(a) Conception and design of the trial, or analysis and interpretation of the data;
(b) Drafting or revising the article critically for important intellectual content;
(c) Final approval of the version to be published.

Declaration of Helsinki

This deals with the setting up of a trial and is principally intended for the protection of the participants.

- Moral and scientific justification for study
- Carried out by scientifically qualified persons working under medical supervision
- Consideration of scientific benefit to subject risk ratio
- Risk of alteration to subject personality is usually unacceptable, for example by use of hallucinogenic drugs
- Consent of subjects
- Protection of subjects

AUDIT

Audit is the systematic peer review of all areas of clinical practice with the object of maintaining and improving the quality of that practice; 'the systematic and critical analysis of the quality of clinical care... the associated use of resources and the resulting outcome and quality of life for the patient'. (NHSME: Clinical Audit: Meeting and improving standards of healthcare).

Research is the discipline of improving medical care by expanding the known areas of medical science, whereas audit is monitoring practice within those known areas.

Publications can be obtained both through audit and research. Audit rarely involves a departure from accepted clinical practice and doesn't have a control group. Hence ethics committee approval is rarely needed for audit projects.

The audit loop

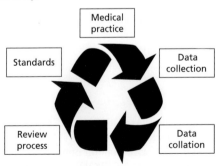

'It has long been a cornerstone of anaesthetic practice in the UK that our actions should be held up to our peers for regular review.' Graham 1992.

Confidential enquiry into maternal deaths

Beecher and Todd, 1952. This has reported every 3 years since then, and is the longest-established medical audit project. It considers maternal death up to 42 days postpartum. Since 1984 this has considered the whole UK. There is a considerable time delay between the information gathering and the publication of the report.

The recent report dealt with the years 1997–1999. The rate was 11.4 deaths per 100,000 maternities. The causes are:

- Thrombosis and thromboembolism, which account for 33% of all direct maternal deaths (DMD).
- Hypertensive disease of pregnancy remains the second leading cause of direct deaths.
- Sepsis.
- Deaths in early pregnancy.
- Amniotic fluid embolism.
- Haemorrhage.

Anaesthesia: There were three deaths attributed to anaesthesia, an increase on the one case in the last report, although still only accounting for 3% of DMD. The one death was due to anaesthesia for Caesarean section, and the two others were deaths in patients on intensive care after numerous interventions. A key recommendation was that anaesthetists were unaware of the dangers of hypotension caused by oxytocin in hypovolaemic patients.

Confidential enquiry into perioperative deaths (CEPOD)

1956: Association of Anaesthetists of Great Britain and Ireland: Considered 1,000 cases.
1987: CEPOD: Dealt with London only.
1989: National CEPOD (NCEPOD) 1: England and Wales, sample only.
1990: NCEPOD 2: E&W, NI, Guernsey, Isle of Man, Jersey.

1993: NCEPOD 3: This, and all subsequent reports, addressed deaths within 30 days of surgery. It emphasised shortages of emergency theatres and ITU facilities.

1995: NCEPOD 4: This report concentrated on age 6–70, and was the largest so far, with 19,816 reports.

1999: 'Extremes of age'. This emphasised the need for paediatric specialism.

2001: 'Changing the way we operate'. Discussed multidisciplinary audit, gaps in provision between high-dependency unit (HDU) and wards, and importance of CVP monitoring.

2002: 'Functioning as a team?' Recommends more ITU sessions, deplores the absence of monitoring, and once again recommends more post-mortem examinations.

The law and equipment

Electrical safety

Macroshock: At 5 mA there will be pain, at 50 mA paralysis, at 100 mA ventricular fibrillation (VF).

Microshock: This occurs via an intracardiac catheter, for example a central line; just 0.1 mA can cause VF.

HTM (Health technical memorandum) II, 1977: This deals with antistatic precautions, and these being allowed to lapse.

Electromed: Classes

I	Earthed
IIA	No exposed metal earthed
IIB	Double insulated
	Types
BF	external surgery
CF	Cardiac; lower current leakage

Diathermy: What the words mean
- *Coagulation:* Pulsed current
- *Cutting:* Continuous current
- *Bipolar:* 40 W delivered
- *Monopolar:* 150–400 W delivered

Suction

Features: Valve, gauge (anticlockwise), filter with cut-off valve to prevent contamination of central reservoir, collecting reservoir with antifoaming agent.

Standards: (For anaesthetic purposes); 10 sec to generate -500 mmHg with displacement capacity of 25 l/min. Tubing needs to have low resistance and low compliance.

Scavenging

The threshold of smell is 33 parts per million (ppm). N_2O is a greenhouse gas, it depresses methionine synthese and causes abortion (Cohen), although this is contentious. Volatiles are HCFCs (not CFCs) and have minimal effect on the ozone layer.

Control of substances hazardous to health (COSHH) 1988

It is a criminal offence not to apply this act since the lifting of crown immunity. It sets requirements for alternatives to mask anaesthesia, named manager with responsibility for implementation, closed system filling for vaporisers to be carried out in a fume cupboard, and minimum rates of air supply:

Operating theatres	$0.65\,m^3/s$
Anaesthetic rooms	$0.15\,m^3/s$
Preparation rooms	$0.1\,m^3/s$
Recovery	15 air changes per hour.

It also lays down time weighted average exposure levels for volatiles, to be monitored by the use of personal samplers to be carried within the breathing area of the practitioner. These are:

N_2O	100 ppm (USA: 25 ppm)
Isoflurane	50 ppm
Enflurane	20 ppm
Halothane	10 ppm
(USA, for all volatiles, limit is 2 ppm)	

Other methods

Activated charcoal: Cardiff aldasorber; weighs 1 kg when new. Takes up volatiles not N_2O.

Soda-lime: Consists of 90% CaOH, 5% NaOH, 1% KOH and silicate (to form granules), moisture and an indicator. Takes up CO_2, produces moisture and heat. There is a risk of degradation of volatiles by dry soda-lime, to produce toxic products.

Active scavenging

Consists of:

- Collecting system (30 mm connections)
- Transfer system (with pressure release valve to prevent barotrauma)
- Disposal system
- Systems should not permit pressure greater than 2 kPa at flows of 90 l/min.

Sterilisation

This can be considered as decontamination, disinfection, and sterilisation. The three are not the same.

1. *Decontamination:* This is the removal of infected matter.
2. *Disinfection:* This is the destruction of organisms but not spores. Methods are:
   - Pasteurisation; water, 70°C for 20 min or 80°C for 10 min; used for plastics.
   - Boiling.
   - Chlorhexidine 0.05% × 30 min; used for skin.
   - Glutaraldehyde 2%; for endoscopes.
   - Sodium hypochlorite 10%; for benches and surfaces.
3. *Sterilisation:* This kills organisms and spores. Methods are:
   - Autoclaving; pressurised steam, 130°C; for instruments and tubes. Indicator paper shows autoclaved wrapping.
   - Dry heat; 160°C; for delicate instruments.
   - Ethylene oxide; for whole machines, only available in specialist centres. It causes pulmonary oedema, so equipment must be left to elute for 10 days.
   - Gamma irradiation; for disposables.

Infection risk to staff

The hazards are from exposure to diseases such as TB, hepatitis B and C, and HIV. The Association of Anaesthetists recommends the wearing of gloves for all procedures where the anaesthetist comes into contact with the patient. Most Trusts now insist on documentary evidence of immunisation against hepatitis B. In the event of a needlestick injury:

- Thoroughly clean the wound site
- Report incident to local manager
- Take blood from patient for hepatitis B (HB) status
- Take blood from victim for HB immune status

If HIV known in patient, offer post-exposure chemoprophylaxis within one hour. If hepatitis B known in patient, offer specific immunoglobulin within 48 h.

If hepatitis C known in patient, repeat serology at 6 weeks and 3 months.

Desert island anaesthesia

If you had to take the minimum of kit to a remote location, what would you choose?

Firstly, some absolute essentials without which you couldn't begin:

- A table, that tilts in such a way that the airway can be cleared.
- A light source, which can be directed at what you are doing.
- A means of applying positive pressure, without necessarily having a source of fresh gas; a self-inflating bag.
- A means of applying suction; a foot-operated portable suction device.
- A skilled assistant.

Thereafter, some specifics:

- *An induction agent for all seasons:* Ketamine, or thiopentone (but you'll need to remember distilled water for preparation). Propofol denatures at altitude.
- *An analgesic:* Morphine.
- *A relaxant:* Vecuronium, which is packaged with water for preparation. Most of the others, including suxamethonium, require a fridge, which you don't have.

- *A local anaesthetic:* Lidocaine 1%.
- *Emergency drugs:* Atropine and adrenaline.
- *Venous access:* 20 G venflons will work for small and large veins.
- *Airway control:* Washable transparent masks, guedel airways and a supply of reusable red-rubber 6 mm cuffed tubes, which will fit children with the cuff up or down, and all adults.

If your Man Friday is resourceful, then have some luxuries:
- Electrical power.
- An oxygen concentrator.
- Sterile saline for intravenous administration.

For monitoring, you have the Mark one digital sensor and eyeball combination. Good luck!

History

It was a circus showman, Horace Wells, who first (albeit unsuccessfully) demonstrated nitrous oxide; its discovery is attributed to Sir Humphrey Davy. The next player in the history of anaesthesia, William Morton, is usually described as a dentist. However, there is no evidence that he qualified in either dentistry or medicine; he made money from dodgy real estate dealings and from the use of ether for the painless fitting of false teeth. Morton was, in short, also a maverick; however, he probably did give the first ether anaesthetic in Boston, Massachusetts on October 16th 1846. This was replicated in Gower Street, London, on 19th December by James Robinson (who was a dentist) at the behest of Francis Boott, who had heard of events in Boston by letter. On the 21st December, just two days later, at University College Hospital a medical student called William Squire provided either anaesthesia for Robert Liston to cut the leg off an unfortunate Frederick Churchill, who was a butler. The second anaesthetic, Squire's, is often (and mistakenly) given the accolade of the first UK anaesthetic although this belongs rightly to Robinson.

Moving on to Vienna in 1884, Sigmund Freud suggested to his friend Karl Koller that cocaine might have therapeutic properties. He went on to become very wealthy indeed when he discovered that cataract extraction was the first complex major that could be done in 20 min.

John Snow was probably the first doctor of what is now known as public health medicine although it is in anaesthesia that his place in history rightly belongs. Just as Morton is associated with ether, so is Snow associated with chloroform, famously, in the case of Queen Victoria and the birth of Prince Leopold in 1853. The impact this had on obstetric practice was not as great as has been reported and would undoubtedly have disappointed Snow. Then as now, the obstetrician was eager to blame obstetric complications on anaesthesia – Dr Locock, Victoria's attending obstetrician, thought that the chloroform prolonged the intervals between pains, and 'retarded labour somewhat'.

Pearl Harbor produced the greatest urban myth in the history of anaesthesia, when it was widely held that injudicious use of thiopentone in hypovolaemia was responsible for the death of many thousands of American servicemen. Whereas in fact their deaths were attributable to the Japanese Navy and Air Force.

Griffiths' use of curare (Intercostrin) in 1942 meant that patients no longer required extreme depths of anaesthesia for the conduct of major surgery. Previous attempts at the use of intercostrin, resulting in the overnight manual ventilation of patients by Prof Rovenstine and his assistant Papper at Columbia Medical School, had been largely unsuccessful to the point where it had been discarded as 'too dangerous for use'. Many trainees in anaesthesia would recognise the inconvenience of prolonged manual ventilation but might point out that attention to detail in dosage terms was all that had been required.

The history of anaesthesia is punctuated by the development of drugs whose ultimate use would have surprised their inventors. Etomidate, for example, was a 17β-hydroxylase inhibitor with purely incidental hypnotic qualities. However it was not until etomidate was used for sedation on ITU that its full lethal potential was discovered. Similarly pethidine, a synthetic anticholinergic, was found to have coincidental, but weak, properties inhibiting C-fibre transmission. From then on pethidine became a favourite substance of misuse among midwives, whose mistaken belief in their status as 'independent practitioners' was perpetrated by their unsupervised use of this largely useless drug.

More prolonged manual ventilation illustrates our short and irreverent history. Now in Copenhagen, and this time by medical students in 1952 and during an epidemic of anterior poliomyelitis. Although intermittent positive pressure ventilation (IPPV) had been used at an earlier time than this, here is the first description of IPPV that a contemporary anaesthetist would recognise.

Suckling had already developed halothane in 1951 but it was not until 1956 that it entered clinical use. The initial improvement in quality of anaesthesia provided by halothane was never greatly improved upon by the subsequent development of the other volatile anaesthetics.

The last developments in anaesthesia in the 20th century would be the laryngeal mask airway and diisopropyl phenol, or propofol. The two go together, not just in chronological terms, both appearing in the 1980s – but also because it was the reflex-suppressant properties of propofol that allowed successful placement of laryngeal mask airways. So ended the era of prolonged airway maintenance by mask and airway, and a new era of anaesthesia where record taking and continuous monitoring gained supremacy.

The business plan

This may be set out as below.
- *Mission statement:* Specific to provision of anaesthetic services, but consistent with the Mission Statement of the Trust.
- *Aims and objectives*
- *Service capacity:*
  - Organisation and management.
  - *Staffing:* Consultants, university posts, trainees, research staff, career grades, non-medical and administrative staff.
  - *Facilities:* Theatres, ITU, pain clinics, office space, laboratory, library, teaching space, computers, accommodation.

- Allocation of time, Programmed Activities (PA), expressed as whole time equivalents (WTE). Also commitment to committee work and teaching.
- *Utilisation:* Activity tables for previous year; Korner data.
  - Cases, hours, and breakdown by speciality and NCEPOD categories.
  - ITU
  - Obstetrics
  - Chronic pain
  - Acute pain
  - Resus and A&E activities
  - Teaching
  - Special interests
- Financial resources
- *SWOT:* Strengths, Weaknesses, Opportunities, Threats: *PEST* (Political, Economical, Sociological, Technological)
- *Aims and objectives:* For the following year.

Risk management

This is the management of an unexpected adverse event befalling a patient under anaesthetic care anywhere in the hospital. The objects are to limit damage, prevent recurrence, and protect the clinician and department from litigation.

- Clinical director notified.
- Second clinician assumes care of patient.
- Clinician involved completes factual account of events.
- Spokesman appointed for liaison with family of patient; family informed.
- All documentation photocopied.
- Medical defence organisations involved.
- Systematic investigation, if appropriate, to determine causation, and prevent repetition.

Reporting adverse reactions

Adverse reactions should be reported to The Committee on Safety of Medicines, London SW8 5BR using the Yellow Card scheme. With newer drugs, (denoted with an inverted triangle in data sheets and in the British National Formulary) all reactions should be reported. With established drugs, serious suspected reactions should be notified.

Adroit = Adverse reactions on-line reporting system.
Phone numbers:
- *CSM London:* 0800 731 6789
- *CSM Mersey:* 0151 794 8206
- *CSM Wales:* 029 2074 4181
- *CSM Northern:* 0191 232 1525
- *CSM West Midlands:* 0121 507 5672

(See also Management of Allergic Reactions, in Resuscitation and Critical Incident Management Section)

Internet bookmarks

Societies and Associations
- Difficult Airway Society
  http://www.das.mailbox.co.uk
- The Association of Anaesthetists
  http://www.aagbi.org
- Society for Computing & Technology in Anaethesia
  http://www.scata.org.uk
- The Royal Society of Medicine
  http://www.roysocmed.ac.uk

Colleges
- Royal College of Anaesthetists
  http://www.rcoa.ac.uk
- The Royal College of Surgeons of England
  http://www.rcseng.ac.uk
- The Royal College of Surgeons of Edinburgh
  http://www.rcsed.ac.uk

Information
- ExPASy – Biochemical Pathways
  http://www.expasy.org/cgi-bin/search-biochem-index
- Gray's Anatomy of the Human Body
  http://www.bartleby.com/107

- National electronic Library for Health
  http://www.nelh.nhs.uk
- PubMed Medline
  http://www.ncbi.nlm.nih.gov
- OMNI
  http://omni.ac.uk
- On-line Medical Dictionary
  http://cancerweb.ncl.ac.uk/omd
- British National Formulary
  http://www.bnf.org
- British pharmacopoeia
  http://www.pharmacopoeia.org.uk

Government and Regulation
- GMC
  http://www.gmc-uk.org
- Department of Health
  http://www.doh.gov.uk
- The National Health Service
  http://www.nhs.uk
- NHS Direct Online
  http://www.nhsdirect.nhs.uk
- Audit Commission
  http://www.audit-commission.gov.uk
- Commission for Health Improvement
  http://www.chi.nhs.uk
- NICE
  http://www.nice.org.uk
- National Confidential Enquiry into Perioperative Deaths
  http://www.ncepod.org.uk

Insurance
- The Medical Defence Union
  http://www.the-mdu.com
- Medical Protection Society
  http://www.medicalprotection.org

Evidence
- Netting The Evidence
  http://www.sheffield.ac.uk/~scharr/ir/netting

- Bandolier Evidence based health care
  http://www.jr2.ox.ac.uk/bandolier

Journals
- nature.com
  http://www.nature.com
- The New England Journal of Medicine
  http://content.nejm.org
- The Lancet
  http://www.thelancet.com

Working in the UK
- The British Council
  http://www.britishcouncil.org/index.htm
- The Plab Course
  http://www.plab.co.uk
- GMC & PLAB
  http://www.gmc-uk.org/register/plab.htm
- IELTS – International English Language Testing System –
  What is IELTS
  http://www.ielts.org
- West Suffolk Hospitals NHS Trust
  http://www.wsufftrust.org.uk
- Greenwich Medical Media
  http://www.greenwich-medical.co.uk

INITIATION OF INTENSIVE CARE

The ICU admission

The skill is to exclude or treat medical emergencies first, as you will be amazed what gets missed and under treated. Assume all previous teams have no idea how to fully resuscitate a patient. The use of this scheme will avoid the omission of any detail in the admission of a patient to the Intensive Care Unit or in the subsequent management.

Admission

Emergency or elective admission/age/gender
Past medical history and drug history/allergy/addiction: Surgical cases: Any drugs up to and including morning of operation?

If admission is the result of trauma:
Mechanism and time of injury/velocity/restrained?
Vital signs at scene/scores/others injured.

Anaesthetic time/operation/complications.
Blood loss/fluid replacement/urine output perioperatively.
Lines *in situ*/urinary catheter.
Airway/ventilation figures/FiO_2.

Specific requirements: Inotropes/antibiotics/DVT prophylaxis/feeding.

Examination and review

- Top of sheet: Date/day number/temperature
- *CNS:* Glasgow coma scale (GCS)/AVPU/localising signs/ mental state
- *CVS:* BP/heart rate/heart sounds/central pressures/output studies/PaO_2 on what FiO_2
- *RS:* Airway/breath sounds/drains
- *GI:* Feeding/aspirate/sounds/drains
- *GU:* Input/output/balance
- *Host defence:* Includes temperature, leucocyte count and microbiology cultures

- *Skin:* Integrity of pressure areas
- *Musculoskeletal:* Tone and bulk

Standard monitoring
Oximetry, ECG, CVP, respiratory rate, $etCO_2$, HR, IBP/NIBP, UO, hourly fluid balance, sedation score, pain score, GCS, temperature $\pm$ CO.

Investigations
Not all will be necessary every day. They are grouped together in as logical a manner as possible.
- FBC/U&E/LFT/Ca^+/Mg^+/Amylase/Clotting/D-dimer/Trace elements/CRP
- Blood sugar
- CXR/ECG
- ABG (state FiO_2), lactate
- 24 h and dipsticked urine/creatinine clearance/osmolalities
- Microbiology: Hepatitis A, B, C and HIV status/swabs/sputum/blood cultures/urines/line cultures
- Pregnancy test: Do not make assumptions about unknown, unconscious female patients
- Blood products available

Treatment
- Ventilation: V_E/mean airway pressure/FiO_2; CPAP/ASB/NIPPV; Physiotherapy
- Sedation/analgesia/paralysis (rarely needed)
- Fluids/Feeding $\pm$ insulin (enteral feeds as soon as feasible)
- Gastric mucosal protection, nasogastric tube
- Position: Head up/rotating mattress/use of prone position
- DVT prophylaxis
- Antibiotics (state number of days)
- Inotropic support
- Filtration/dialysis/plasma exchange

Drugs you may consider
- Sedatives
- Analgesics
- Low molecular weight heparin (LMWH)

- Antibiotics
- Sucralfate/H_2 blocker/proton pump inhibitor
- Insulin
- Inotropes
- Potassium

Ward round and plan
- Persons present on ward round
- Major events in last 24 h
- Plan for today/for next few days
- Review drug and fluid charts
- Ultimate objective
- Explanation given to relatives

Practicalities of ventilators and ventilation

Classification of ventilators
- *Hunter 1961:* Divided into volume pre-set and pressure pre-set
- *Mapleson 1962:* Flow generated ventilators (FGV) or pressure generated ventilators (PGV)
- *Ward 1973:* Low-powered or high-powered;
  - Mechanical thumbs
  - Minute volume dividers
  - Bag squeezers
  - Intermittent blowers
- *Inspiration:* Pressure/time graphs are straight lines with FGV but curves with PGV

Inspiratory-expiratory change (cycling)
By volume, flow, pressure or time.

Expiration
Positive pressure can be applied as resistance to expiration positive end expiratory Pressure (PEEP).

Expiratory-inspiratory change
Can be patient triggered, or by time or by volume, i.e. when bellows are full.

When to intubate

The commonest reason is to facilitate ventilation. This can be further broken down as follows:

- To protect the upper airway; shared airway, trauma, unstable fractures
- To protect the lower airway; risk of soiling from gastric contents
- When paralysis is required for surgery

When to ventilate

- Acute respiratory insufficiency or arrest
- Respiratory failure refractory to increased FiO_2 and other measures
- Progressive accumulation of CO_2
- Mechanical compromise, e.g. flail chest
- Intubation, if prolonged

Indications for tracheostomy

- To bypass obstruction above the level of the trachea
- To separate passage of food and air
- To permit repeated aspiration of secretions
- To allow comfortable prolonged or long-term ventilation

How to ventilate

Start with minimum intervention and increase as necessary, i.e.:

- Face mask
- Continuous positive airway pressure (CPAP)
- Intubation and ventilation with biphasic positive airways pressure (BIPAP)

PEEP is usually required in ITU settings. If BIPAP is unsatisfactory, consider controlled ventilation.

Setting up BIPAP

BIPAP is now the most popular form of ventilation on ITU.

- Set pressures at $20/5\,cmH_2O$ at a rate of 12–15/min, to achieve V_T of 10–15 ml/kg
- The lower pressure (effectively, PEEP) can be increased if the lungs are stiff in order to improve alveolar recruitment

- Mean airway pressure should be minimized to prevent barotrauma, and peak pressure should not exceed $40\,cmH_2O$ in any event; a lower V_T (10–15 ml/kg) should prevent volutrauma
- Start with FiO_2 at 1.0 and reduce to lowest level that keeps SpO_2 acceptable, i.e. above 92%

Adjustment Of BIPAP

Think of manipulating three parameters:

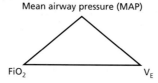

Mean airway pressure (MAP)

FiO_2 V_E

$V_E = V_T \times f$

V_T = Inspiratory flow rate $\times$ inspiratory time

f = 60/(inspiratory time + expiratory time)

Mean airway pressure is proportional to:
- Compliance
- PEEP
- I:E ratio – which is usually 1:2 but may be 1:1 or even 2:1

Air trapping

This occurs when inspiration encroaches on expiration. It results in defective gas exchange and possibly in barotrauma. The pattern of ventilation will have to be altered.

Sedation

All units have their favourite cocktails, usually a combination of anaesthesia (propofol), sedative (midazolam) and opiate (morphine/fentanyl/remifentanil). Start with e.g. propofol infusion + morphine midazolam (M&M) boluses. Review daily in view of patient's physiological status, sedation, ventilation and analgesia needs. Sedation score 2 h and consider sedation 'hold' daily.

Withdrawal of ventilatory support

The weaning process is a reversal of the cascade of support, from most interventional to least. Patient must be able to manage each step for an appropriate period of time.

- Reduction of sedation and reversal of paralysis
- On BIPAP, reduce FiO_2 and pressures in a progressive fashion. This means that the patient has to do progressively more of the work of breathing
- Change BIPAP to assisted spontaneous breathing (ASB)
- Change to CPAP often by increasing periods; may need to ventilate formally overnight, for example
- From CPAP onto T-Piece or tracheostomy mask

When to extubate

Is the condition, for which the patient was intubated, better?

Criteria:
- Cardiovascular and metabolic stability
- Protection of airway
- PaO_2 >9 kPa on FiO_2 <0.4
- Vital capacity >15 ml/kg, with ability to increase it voluntarily
- Respiratory rate <20/min, which does not increase when support is withdrawn

Replacement of defective tracheal tube

- Sedate, paralyse if necessary and increase FiO_2 to preoxygenate
- Change to self-inflating bag from ventilator
- Laryngoscopy, suction, aspirate nasogastric tube
- Cuff leak test: Deflate cuff, leak indicates presence of adequate lumen for new tube
- Pass bougie down existing tube
- Change tube over bougie

Cardiorespiratory manipulation

Acute respiratory distress syndrome (ARDS): definition
- Identifiable acute lung injury

- Normal albumin
- PCWP <15
- Decreased compliance
- Increased shunt
- Divide PaO_2 (mmHg)/FiO_2: 150–300 implies injury, <150 indicates ARDS
- CXR demonstrates bilateral infiltrates

Goal-directed therapy

This comes and goes as a fashion. The relationship between DO_2 and VO_2 is complex in critical illness and in different types of condition. The classic work by Shoemaker suggests the following is beneficial in young trauma patients, but would be unrealistic in a 90 year old.

Cardiac index (CI)	150% of normal; >4.5 l/min/m^2
DO_2	>600 ml/min/m^2
VO_2	130% of normal; >170 ml/min/m^2
Blood volume	500 ml more than normal

West Suffolk 'what to do in the middle of the night' parameters

Patients must be fully resuscitated first. These are general guidelines – put brain in gear for individual patients!

Haemoglobin	Between 7 and 10 g/dl	Use blood. In cardiac insufficiency, aim for 10.
CI	>2.2 l/min/m^2	Adrenaline (epinephrine)
Systemic vascular resistance index (SVRI)	>1,200 dyne-sec/cm^2/m^2	Noradrenaline (norepinephrine)
PCWP	12–15 cmH$_2$0*	
CVP	12 cmH$_2$0	

* Measure with ventilator disconnected.

If you need a vasodilator, use GTN.

Fluids
- Replace what is being lost e.g. blood
- Because of leaky capillaries, don't overuse crystalloid
- Give boluses of modified starch solution to achieve cardio-vascular parameters
- Gelatins are useful but short lived
- Albumin is the spawn of the devil

Haemodynamic decision making

There are different methods of measuring parameters – the PA catheter has its users and abusers, as does the Doppler, the bioimpedance thing that no-one ever uses and so on. SiO_2 monitoring has its champions also. However, by knowledge of CI and wedge pressure:

	PAWP <18	PAWP >18
CI >2.2	I Normality: No action required	III Diuretic + Vasodilator
CI <2.2	II Volume	IV Inotropic Support + Vasodilator

Infection on ITU

Sepsis syndrome

It is important if sepsis is suspected to get a baseline C-reactive protein (CRP), which is a marker of bacterial infection.

Diagnosis is based on:
- Fever over 38.3°C or hypothermia less than 35.6°C
- Tachycardia greater than 90 bpm
- Tachypnoea over 20 bpm or requiring ventilation
- *Hypotension:* Systolic blood pressure less than 90 mmHg or having fallen by 40 mmHg, or two of:
  - Unexplained metabolic acidosis with BE greater than −5 mmol/l
  - Acute renal failure (ARF) with urine output below 0.5 ml/kg/h
  - Impaired cognition

- Arterial hypoxaemia
- Coagulopathy
- CI over 4.0 with SVRI less than 1,400

Other strategies for managing sepsis may include steroids, methylene blue, activated protein C, early haemofiltration or the latest ICU fad.

Prevention of secondary infection is vital and should include:
- Handwashing before/after/between
- Staff aprons and gloves
- Line change policy
- Closed suction
- Patient isolation
- 1:1 nursing
- Enteral rather than parenteral feeding

Keeping MRSA-infested orthopaedic surgeons out is desirable but not usually possible, as they are almost certainly bigger than you.

The following antibiotic regimes are suggestions only. Definitive therapy depends on culture and sensitivity. While waiting for this, most units have guidelines for specific situations.

Line infection: Flucloxacillin 0.25–1.0 g qds + fucidin 580 mg tds or gentamicin 3–7 mg/kg od.

Intra-abdominal infection: Metronidazole 500 mg tds + cefotaxime 1–2 g tds ± gentamicin 7 mg/kg daily.

Community acquired pneumonia: We use ceftriaxone 1 g daily and clarithromycin 500 mg bd.

Nosocomial pneumonia: Flucloxacillin + cefotaxime.

Meningococcal septicaemia: Benzylpenicillin 2.4 g every 4–6 h, or cefotaxime 1 g tds.

Other meningitis: Ceftazidime 1 g tds or meropenem 1 g tds.

Infective endocarditis: Gentamicin + benzylpenicillin or ampicillin, + flucloxacillin if *Staph. aureus* possible.

Neutropenic patients: Piperacillin + gentamicin + antifungal after 3 days (fluconazole 1–2 mg/kg/d)

Total blind therapy: Flucloxacillin + cefotaxime + metronidazole

Second line agents: Ceftazidime 1–2 g bd
Ciprofloxacin 200 mg bd
Imipenem 1–2 g/d divided doses
Teicoplanin 400 mg, then 200 mg/d
Vancomycin 500 mg qds
Aztreonam 1–2 g tds
Amphotericin 0.25–1.0 mg/kg/d

Management of acute poisoning

- *Resuscitation*
- *Cannulation* and samples to lab for immediate assay of paracetamol and salicylate levels; retain serum for toxicology
- *History,* from Paramedics and relatives. Do not trust the patient
- *Empty stomach* (not in case of paraffin or corrosive ingestion–risk of aspiration) and instillation of activated charcoal (even in delayed presentation, as it may interrupt enterohepatic circulation of drugs). Leave in a nasogastric tube. Repeated charcoal instillation is useful for drugs with a small volume of distribution but long $t_{1/2}$, such as barbiturates, theophylline, digoxin and salicylates
- *Secondary survey:* CXR, ABG, catheter, CO level
- *Specific antidotes:*

β-blockers	Atropine, isoprenaline, glucagon
CO	Hyperbaric O_2 ($t_{1/2}$ of COHb is 250 min in air, 50 min in 100% O_2, and 22 min at 2.5 bar)
Cyanide	Dicobalt edetate 20 ml i.v. chelates CN, Na thiosulphate 50 ml 25% presents sulphur substrate for enzyme
Opioids	Naloxone
Benzodiazepines	Flumazenil
Paracetamol	N-acetylcysteine
Digoxin	Dig-specific Fab antibody fragments (digibind)

(table continued)

Metals	Chelating agents: Desferrioxamine, dimercaprol, penicillamine
Organophosphorus	Atropine, oximes, pyridostigmine (used for prophylaxis)
Ethylene glycol	Ethanol
Sympathomimetics	β-blockers
Phenothiazines	Benztropine
Anticholinergics	Physostigmine
Oxidising agents	Methylene blue

- Specific measures: e.g. pacing in tricyclic toxicity
- Diuresis or dialysis: Keep urinary pH over 6.5 to prevent myoglobin deposition. Mannitol is better than frusemide. For dialysis to be effective, the toxin must have a small Vd_{ss}, and minimal protein binding. For dialysis, it must be of low molecular weight; for filtration, it must have a high affinity for the adsorbent. There is no point in either measure if the extracorporeal clearance is exceeded by the endogenous clearance of the substance

National phone numbers of poisons units: 0870 600 6266

Dialysis

In ARF, urea rises by 5 mmol/l/day and creatinine by 15 μmol/l/day. Most would advocate dialysis at 30 mmol/l urea. Only drugs present in plasma can be eliminated by dialysis, thus must be water soluble and with a small volume of distribution. Lipid soluble drugs may be eliminated by haemofiltration, allowing longer equilibration between compartments.

Peritoneal dialysis (PD)

Uses: Treatment of ARF, chronic renal failure (CRF); cooling in hyperpyrexia.

Requirements: Insertion of silastic Tenchkoff catheter into peritoneum inferior to the umbilicus in the midline.

Method: Instil 1,000 ml dialysate with 500 u heparin at body temperature (unless hyperpyrexial), dwell 30 minutes, drain over 30 minutes; one cycle = one hour. Composition of dialysate, in terms of osmolality and potassium especially, is dictated by the condition.

Advantages: Simpler than other modes, better for children. Safer with bleeding problems than other modes. Relatively inexpensive. The most cardiovascularly stable method.

Disadvantages: Slow elimination of toxins and excess fluids, therefore inappropriate in highly catabolic states. Needs intact peritoneum. Relatively contraindicated in ventilated patients, and in respiratory distress. Peritonitis is a risk.

Haemodialysis (HD)

Uses: Treatment of ARF, CRF; elimination of poisons; correction of fluid overload.

Requirements: Arterial and large-bore venous access. Dialysis machine which presents the blood to a membrane adjacent to the dialysate (see PD).

Method: Formation of shunt (often at wrist) or separate arterial and venous cannulae, priming of machine, heparin infusion 1,000 u/h.

Advantages: More rapid elimination of toxins and fluid than PD.

Disadvantages: Access, expense, bleeding, aluminium toxicity, removal of vitamins and water-soluble nutrients. Air embolus, haemolysis.

Continuous veno-venous haemofiltration (CVVH)

Uses: Treatment of ARF, CRF; elimination of poisons; correction of fluid overload.

Requirements: Double large-bore venous access. Blood pump and bubble trap. Filter. No dialysate required.

Method: Access, priming pump and filter, heparin.

Advantages: Does not divert cardiac output.

Disadvantages: Access, expense, bleeding, removal of vitamins and water-soluble nutrients. Air embolus, haemolysis.

Continuous arterio-venous haemofiltration (CAVH)

Uses: Treatment of ARF, CRF; elimination of poisons; correction of fluid overload.

Requirements: Arterial and large-bore venous access. Filter.

Method: Access, priming of filter, heparin.

Advantages: No pump required.

Disadvantages: Diverts up to 250 ml/min of cardiac output and may precipitate hypotension and hypoperfusion. Tends to clot if mean airway pressure (MAP) not high enough. Access, bleeding, removal of vitamins and water-soluble nutrients. Air embolus.

Haemodiafiltration

Uses: Treatment of ARF, CRF; elimination of poisons; correction of fluid overload.

Requirements: Double large-bore venous access. Blood pump and bubble trap. Filter. Employs countercurrent mechanism exposing dialysate to filter.

Method: Access, priming pump and filter, run through dialysate, heparin.

Advantages: Very efficient. As with veno-venous, no cardiac shunt.

Disadvantages: Access, expense, bleeding, removal of vitamins and water-soluble nutrients. Air embolus, haemolysis.

Haemoperfusion

Uses: Elimination of poisons, severe hepatic failure.

Requirements: Double large-bore venous access, pump, adsorption circuit (amberlite resin or activated charcoal) and heparin.

Method: Access, priming, heparin.

Advantages: In elimination of lipid-soluble and protein-bound toxins, such as barbiturates, tricyclics, paracetamol, salicylates, paraquat, aminophylline and organophosphorus compounds.

Disadvantages: Access, expense, bleeding, haemolysis, thrombocytopenia. Inappropriate for ARF. Does not remove excess fluid as efficiently as other methods.

Pacemakers

Pacemakers are common in elderly patients, who will have ischaemic heart disease.

Pacemaker coding
This is presented as a series of 3 or 5 letters; for example, VVI is ventricle paced, ventricle sensed, inhibited.

I Chamber paced; ventricle, atrium, dual.

II Chamber sensed; V, A, D, none.

III Mode of response; triggered, inhibited, dual, none, reverse.

IV Programmable functions; P = simple programmable, M = multi xprogrammable, C = communicating, 0 = none.

V Antidysrhythmia function; bursts, normal rate competition, scanning, external.

Suxamethonium may cause inappropriate inhibition.

Diathermy may deprogramme the pacemaker or may set up induced current in the wire if current is parallel to it, destroying the box or injuring the myocardium, increasing the threshold.

Magnets, although they may convert VVI to VOO (fixed rate) may also deprogramme sophisticated pacemakers.

Temporary pacing: Indications
- Complete heart block
- Second degree heart block: Symptomatic type I, any type II
- Symptomatic first degree block
- Trifascicular block; any AV block with two other conduction defects, or alternating RBBB/LBBB

Temporary pacing: Method
Right internal jugular cannulation, with X-ray screening for sitting of wire, and lignocaine cover if ventricle is irritable. Increase voltage until capture of ventricular contraction

occurs, indicating threshold. An initial threshold of <1 volt at 1 ms pulse width is preferable. Set on double this threshold, check daily for increase.

Bronchoscopy

This is how to record what you have done.
- *Set up:* Instrument used/indication
- *Preparation:* Position/pre-oxygenation/suction/sedation
- *Portal:* Oral/nasal endotracheal or tracheostomy tube
- *Findings:* Trachea/carina/mucosa/main bronchi/bronchus intermedius/lobar bronchi; blood/secretions/plugs/sputum/foreign material
- *Procedure:* Lavage/suction/brushings/biopsy
- *Post-procedure:* O_2/ventilation/position

Transfers

Checklist
- Experienced attendants
- Equipment
  - Transfer pack(s) checked with good knowledge of contents.
  - Sufficient quantities of appropriate drugs available, including fridge drugs
  - Emergency airway equipment and self-inflating bag easily to hand
- Mobile phone with charged battery and relevant phone numbers programmed
- Sufficient oxygen $\pm$ cylinder key
- Batteries checked – back-up power cables
- Ambulance service aware/ready
- Bed confirmed and receiving hospital ready
- Case notes
- X-rays, scans, ECGs and all other results
- Cross-matched blood
- Transfer chart prepared
- Return arrangements confirmed – cash required?
- Relatives informed
- Monitoring attached and functional
- Drugs/pumps/lines/monitor secured

Tips and tricks

It pays to be paranoid about oxygen and power supplies. Always have a self-inflating bag-valve-mask device available. Try to keep your hands free to cope with the disaster. If it can go wrong then it probably will – but when it does go wrong *Don't panic!* The transfer should not be considered as just a therapeutic vacuum – active interventions may be considered. Planning, training and reviews will prevent many problems. Staff should have a minimum of two years experience in their specialty.

Brain death

This is recognised in the UK as being synonymous with death. There are preconditions which have to be established and exclusions to be considered before the diagnosis can be made on the criteria below.

Preconditions
- Apnoeic coma
- Irreversible damage of known cause

Exclusions
Brain death cannot be diagnosed if any of these exist
- Hypothermia below 35°C
- Sedative or hypnotic drugs present
- Acid-base derangement
- Metabolic disorder
- Elevated $PaCO_2$
- Hypotension

Criteria
Performed twice (by convention rather than law) at least 30 min apart, more than 6 h after the event causing death, by 2 doctors. Neither may be from the transplant team and both must have been registered more than 5 years, one being a consultant.
- *Pupils:* Direct and consensual responses: Tests second cranial nerve (CII) and parasympathetics
- *Corneal reflex:* Tests CV & CVII

- *Pain to face:* Tests CV & CVII
- *Doll's eye:* In brain stem death, the eyes stay fixed in sockets: This tests CVIII
- *Caloric test:* 30 ml ice cold water applied to clear meatus: No nystagmus implies brain stem death: Tests CVIII
- *Gag:* Tests CIX & CX
- *Apnoea:* Set FiO_2 to 1.0, then disconnect, continuing to give O_2 via cannulae at 6 l/min. Brain stem death is likely if no effort after 10 min or $PaCO_2$ rises above 6.6 kPa

The coroner

The following must be reported to the Coroner. It is often wise to discuss a postoperative death, or the death of an intensive care patient, with the coroner or his representative in any case.

- Sudden death not seen by doctor within 14 days
- Murder, suicide
- Drugs, poisons, medical treatment
- Factory accident
- Pension: Industrial, Disability or War
- Alcohol, self neglect
- Infant, foster child
- Following abortion
- In custody or prison
- Road traffic accident

EMERGENCIES

Critical incident recognition and management

All management algorithms commence with basic life support; control of the airway, confirmation of breathing and oxygenation, and support of the circulation. Most then proceed to advanced life support, as follows. Specific measures are listed under each condition. **ALL MANAGEMENT PLANS ASSUME THAT BASIC AND ADVANCED LIFE SUPPORT HAVE BEEN INSTITUTED.** Failed intubation is covered in the Practical Anaesthesia section; poisoning is covered under Intensive Care.

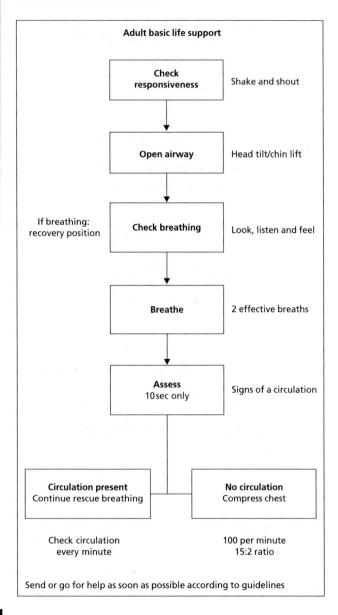

Adult basic life support

| Check responsiveness | Shake and shout |

| Open airway | Head tilt/chin lift |

If breathing: recovery position

| Check breathing | Look, listen and feel |

| Breathe | 2 effective breaths |

| Assess 10 sec only | Signs of a circulation |

| **Circulation present** Continue rescue breathing | **No circulation** Compress chest |

Check circulation every minute

100 per minute
15:2 ratio

Send or go for help as soon as possible according to guidelines

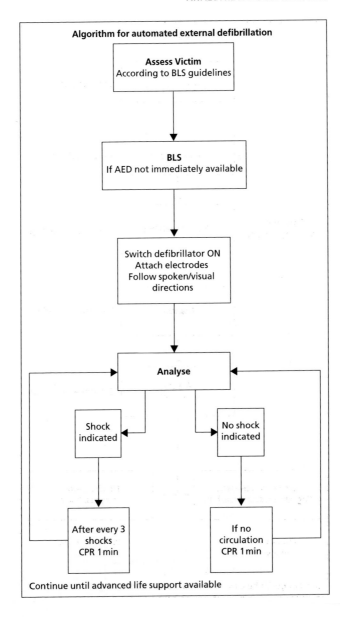

Algorithm for automated external defibrillation

Assess Victim
According to BLS guidelines

↓

BLS
If AED not immediately available

↓

Switch defibrillator ON
Attach electrodes
Follow spoken/visual
directions

↓

Analyse

Shock
indicated

No shock
indicated

After every 3
shocks
CPR 1 min

If no
circulation
CPR 1 min

Continue until advanced life support available

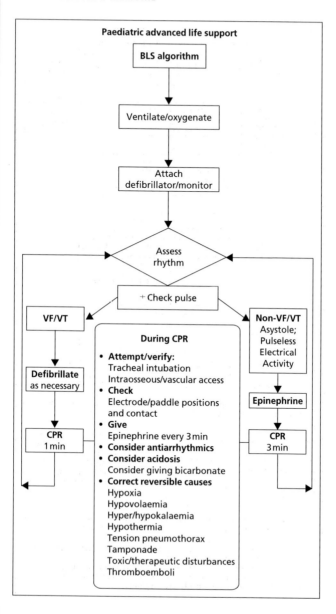

Paediatric advanced life support

BLS algorithm

↓

Ventilate/oxygenate

↓

Attach defibrillator/monitor

↓

Assess rhythm

⁺ Check pulse

VF/VT

↓

Defibrillate as necessary

↓

CPR 1 min

Non-VF/VT Asystole; Pulseless Electrical Activity

↓

Epinephrine

↓

CPR 3 min

During CPR

- **Attempt/verify:** Tracheal intubation Intraosseous/vascular access
- **Check** Electrode/paddle positions and contact
- **Give** Epinephrine every 3 min
- **Consider antiarrhythmics**
- **Consider acidosis** Consider giving bicarbonate
- **Correct reversible causes** Hypoxia Hypovolaemia Hyper/hypokalaemia Hypothermia Tension pneumothorax Tamponade Toxic/therapeutic disturbances Thromboemboli

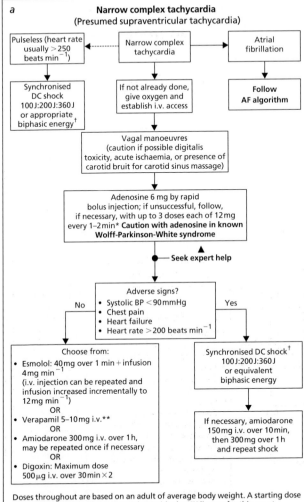

a **Narrow complex tachycardia**
(Presumed supraventricular tachycardia)

Pulseless (heart rate usually >250 beats min^{-1}) ← - - - Narrow complex tachycardia → Atrial fibrillation

Synchronised DC shock 100 J:200 J:360 J or appropriate biphasic energy†

If not already done, give oxygen and establish i.v. access

Follow AF algorithm

Vagal manoeuvres (caution if possible digitalis toxicity, acute ischaemia, or presence of carotid bruit for carotid sinus massage)

Adenosine 6 mg by rapid bolus injection; if unsuccessful, follow, if necessary, with up to 3 doses each of 12 mg every 1–2 min* **Caution with adenosine in known Wolff-Parkinson-White syndrome**

● — Seek expert help

Adverse signs?
• Systolic BP <90 mmHg
• Chest pain
• Heart failure
• Heart rate >200 beats min^{-1}

No   Yes

Choose from:
• Esmolol: 40 mg over 1 min + infusion 4 mg min^{-1} (i.v. injection can be repeated and infusion increased incrementally to 12 mg min^{-1})
  OR
• Verapamil 5–10 mg i.v.**
  OR
• Amiodarone 300 mg i.v. over 1 h, may be repeated once if necessary
  OR
• Digoxin: Maximum dose 500 μg i.v. over 30 min × 2

Synchronised DC shock† 100 J:200 J:360 J or equivalent biphasic energy

If necessary, amiodarone 150 mg i.v. over 10 min, then 300 mg over 1 h and repeat shock

Doses throughout are based on an adult of average body weight. A starting dose of 6 mg adenosine is currently outside the UK licence for this agent.

  * Note 1: Theophylline and related compounds block the effect of adenosine. Patients on dipyridamole, carbamazepine, or with denervated hearts have a markedly exaggerated effect which may be hazardous.
  † Note 2: DC shock is always given under sedation/general anaesthesia.
** Note 3: Not to be used in patients receiving β-blockers.

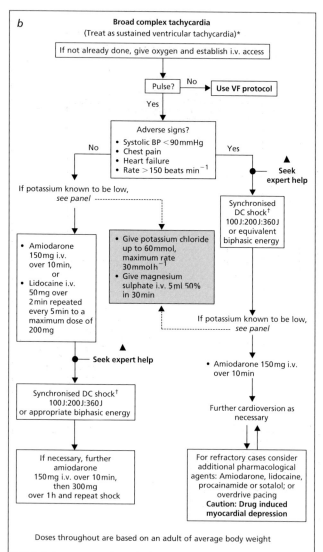

b **Broad complex tachycardia**
(Treat as sustained ventricular tachycardia)*

If not already done, give oxygen and establish i.v. access

Pulse? — No → **Use VF protocol**

Yes

Adverse signs?
• Systolic BP < 90 mmHg
• Chest pain
• Heart failure
• Rate > 150 beats min^{-1}

No ← | → Yes

Seek expert help

If potassium known to be low,
see panel

Synchronised
DC shock†
100 J:200 J:360 J
or equivalent
biphasic energy

• Amiodarone
150 mg i.v.
over 10 min,
or
• Lidocaine i.v.
50 mg over
2 min repeated
every 5 min to a
maximum dose of
200 mg

• Give potassium chloride
up to 60 mmol,
maximum rate
30 mmol h^{-1}
• Give magnesium
sulphate i.v. 5 ml 50%
in 30 min

If potassium known to be low,
see panel

Seek expert help

• Amiodarone 150 mg i.v.
over 10 min

Synchronised DC shock†
100 J:200 J:360 J
or appropriate biphasic energy

Further cardioversion as
necessary

If necessary, further
amiodarone
150 mg i.v. over 10 min,
then 300 mg
over 1 h and repeat shock

For refractory cases consider
additional pharmacological
agents: Amiodarone, lidocaine,
procainamide or sotalol; or
overdrive pacing
**Caution: Drug induced
myocardial depression**

Doses throughout are based on an adult of average body weight

* Note 1: For paroxysms of torsades de pointes, use magnesium as above or
overdrive pacing (expert help strongly recommended).
† Note 2: DC shock is always given under sedation/general anaesthesia.

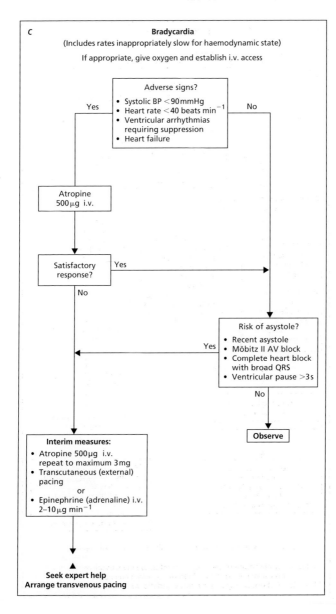

C **Bradycardia**
(Includes rates inappropriately slow for haemodynamic state)

If appropriate, give oxygen and establish i.v. access

Adverse signs?
- Systolic BP <90 mmHg
- Heart rate <40 beats min^{-1}
- Ventricular arrhythmias requiring suppression
- Heart failure

Yes   No

Atropine
500 μg i.v.

Satisfactory response?   Yes

No

Risk of asystole?
- Recent asystole
- Möbitz II AV block
- Complete heart block with broad QRS
- Ventricular pause >3 s

Yes

No

Observe

Interim measures:
- Atropine 500 μg i.v. repeat to maximum 3 mg
- Transcutaneous (external) pacing

or

- Epinephrine (adrenaline) i.v. 2–10 μg min^{-1}

▲
Seek expert help
Arrange transvenous pacing

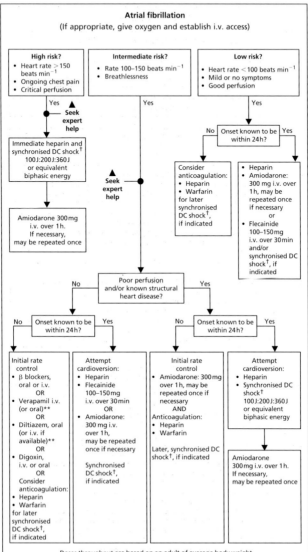

Atrial fibrillation
(If appropriate, give oxygen and establish i.v. access)

High risk?
- Heart rate >150 beats min⁻¹
- Ongoing chest pain
- Critical perfusion

Intermediate risk?
- Rate 100–150 beats min⁻¹
- Breathlessness

Low risk?
- Heart rate <100 beats min⁻¹
- Mild or no symptoms
- Good perfusion

Yes

Seek expert help

Immediate heparin and synchronised DC shock†
100 J:200 J:360 J or equivalent biphasic energy

Amiodarone 300 mg i.v. over 1 h. If necessary, may be repeated once

Yes

Seek expert help

Yes

Onset known to be within 24 h?

No   Yes

Consider anticoagulation:
- Heparin
- Warfarin
for later synchronised DC shock†, if indicated

- Heparin
- Amiodarone: 300 mg i.v. over 1 h, may be repeated once if necessary
  or
- Flecainide 100–150 mg i.v. over 30 min and/or synchronised DC shock†, if indicated

Poor perfusion and/or known structural heart disease?

No   Yes

Onset known to be within 24 h?

No   Yes

Onset known to be within 24 h?

No   Yes

Initial rate control
- β blockers, oral or i.v.
  OR
- Verapamil i.v. (or oral)**
  OR
- Diltiazem, oral (or i.v. if available)**
  OR
- Digoxin, i.v. or oral
  OR
Consider anticoagulation:
- Heparin
- Warfarin
for later synchronised DC shock†, if indicated

Attempt cardioversion:
- Heparin
- Flecainide 100–150 mg i.v. over 30 min
  OR
- Amiodarone: 300 mg i.v. over 1 h, may be repeated once if necessary

Synchronised DC shock†, if indicated

Initial rate control
- Amiodarone: 300 mg over 1 h, may be repeated once if necessary
  AND
Anticoagulation:
- Heparin
- Warfarin

Later, synchronised DC shock†, if indicated

Attempt cardioversion:
- Heparin
- Synchronised DC shock† 100 J:200 J:360 J or equivalent biphasic energy

Amiodarone 300 mg i.v. over 1 h. If necessary, may be repeated once

Doses throughout are based on an adult of average body weight
† Note 1: DC shock is always given under sedation/general anaesthesia.
** Note 2: Not to be used in patients receiving β-blockers.

Newborn life support

Dry the baby, remove any wet cloth and cover

Initial assessment at birth
Start the clock or note the time assess: Colour, Tone, Breathing, Heart Rate

If not breathing ...

Control the airway
Head in the neutral position

Support the breathing
If not breathing – Five inflation breaths (each 2–3 sec duration)
Confirm a response: Increase in Heart Rate or visible Chest Movement

If there is no response
Double check head position and apply Jaw Thrust 5 inflation breaths
Confirm a response: Increase in Heart Rate or visible Chest Movement

If there is *still* no response
- Use a second person (if available) to help with airway control and repeat inflation breaths
- Inspect the oropharynx under direct vision (Is suction needed?) and repeat inflation breaths
- Insert an oropharyngeal (Guedel) airway and repeat inflation breaths
Consider intubation
Confirm a response: Increase in Heart Rate or visible Chest Movement

When the chest is moving
Continue the ventilation breaths if no spontaneous breathing

Check the heart rate
If the heart rate is not detectable *or* slow
(less than around 60 bpm) and *not* increasing

Start chest compressions
First confirm chest movement – if chest not moving *return to airway*
3 chest compressions to 1 breath for 30 sec

Reassess Heart Rate
If improving – stop chest compressions, continue ventilation if not breathing
If heart rate still slow, continue ventilation and chest compressions
Consider venous access and drugs at this stage

At *all* stages, ask ... Do you need help?

In the presence of meconium, remember: Screaming babies: Have an open airway
Floppy babies: Have a look

Airway obstruction

Recognition
a. Cyanosis
b. Paradoxical chest movement
c. Tachycardia

If you can't control an airway, you should be doing something else, like dermatology, perhaps, instead of reading this book.

Malignant hyperpyrexia

Recognition
a. Ca   Myofibril ATPase   Heat 2°C/h
b. Ca   Troponin-C   Rigidity
c. Ca   Phosphorylase kinase   Glycogenolysis

Beware: Family history, young, squints; and the fact that not all the signs may be present. Capnography is the single most useful monitor. It is possible to have had previous uneventful anaesthesia.

Features
Affects 3:1 male:female; associated with squints and musculo-skeletal abnormalities. Autosomal dominant inherited structural abnormality of sarcolemma or sarcoplasmic reticulum. Incidence is 1:200,000 (UK). Diagnosis is based on muscle biopsy, if contracture of 0.2 g occurs in halothane 2% and caffeine 2 mmol/l, this is malignant hyperpyrexia susceptible (MHS). The patient is MH equivocal (MHE) if one or other. MH non-susceptible (MHN) if neither, but the testing is only 95% sensitive. The condition has a 10% mortality.

There is a ryanodine receptor gene, associated with calcium channels in sarcoplasmic reticulum. This is associated, by no means universally, with chromosome 19 q12-13.2.

Management
- Stop trigger agent and stop surgery if possible
- 100% O_2
- Hyperventilate

- Dantrolene (modal effect 2.4 mg/kg, range 1–10 mg/kg)
- Correct acidosis/arrhythmia/hyperkalaemia, encourage diuresis; retain urine for myoglobin assay
- Cool
- Transfer to ITU and monitor progress of condition by serum CK at 6, 12 and 24 h

Morning after diagnosis: Myoglobinuria, and disproportionate rise in plasma CK. Screen proband and family.

Allergic reaction

Recognition
- Cardiovascular: Hypotensive collapse, pulmonary hypertension
- Respiratory: Bronchospasm, oedema
- Skin: Urticaria, oedema, flushing

Beware especially: Suxamethonium, thiopentone, older neuromuscular blocking agents, and the immediate post-induction period.

Definitions
- Intolerance: Qualitatively normal, quantitatively abnormal reaction to drug
- Idiosyncracy: Qualitatively abnormal, but not immunologically-mediated, response to drug
- Anaphylaxis: IgE-mast cell histamine release reaction, type I hypersensitivity
- Anaphylactoid: Direct histamine release from mast cells and macrophages

Management
- Stop administration of suspected agent
- 100% O_2
- ECM if no pulse
- Adrenaline 0.3–1.0 ml of 1:10,000
- Nebulised bronchodilators
- Chlorpheniramine 10 mg
- Steroids; hydrocortisone 100–300 mg

- Plasma expansion 70 ml/kg
- Aminophylline 250 mg over 5 min

Investigation: Blood samples into two EDTA bottles at each of 0, 3, 6, 12 and 24 h after event, store at −25°C, and send to an appropriate laboratory, for trypsin assay which is a marker of mast cell degranulation.

Anaphylactic reactions: Treatment algorithm for adults by first medical responders

Consider when compatible history of severe allergic-type reaction with respiratory difficulty and/or hypotension especially if skin changes present

↓

Oxygen treatment when available

↓

Stridor, wheeze, respiratory distress or clinical signs of shock[1]

↓

Adrenaline (epinephrine)[2,3] 1:1,000 solution 0.5mL (500 μg) i.m.

↓

Repeat in 5 min if no clinical improvement

↓

Antihistamine (chlorphenamine) 10–20 mg i.m./or slow i.v.

↓

In addition

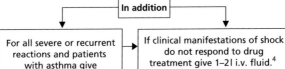

For all severe or recurrent reactions and patients with asthma give Hydrocortisone 100–500 mg i.m./or slowly i.v.

If clinical manifestations of shock do not respond to drug treatment give 1–2 l i.v. fluid.[4] Rapid infusion or one repeat dose may be necessary

[1] An inhaled β$_2$-agonist such as salbutamol may be used as an adjunctive measure if bronchospasm is severe and does not respond rapidly to other treatment.

[2] If profound shock judged **immediately** life threatening give CPR/ALS if necessary. Consider **slow** i.v. adrenaline (epinephrine) 1:10,000 solution. This is **hazardous** and is recommended only for an experienced practitioner who can also obtain i.v. access without delay. Note the different strength of adrenaline (epinephrine) that may be required for i.v. use.

[3] If adults are treated with an Epipen, the 300 μg will usually be sufficient. A second dose may be required. Half doses of adrenaline (epinephrine) may be safer for patients on amitriptyline, imipramine, or β-blocker.

[4] A crystalloid may be safer than a colloid.

January 2002

Amniotic fluid embolus

Recognition: This rare event is said to occur in 'turbulent' vaginal delivery, during operative or instrumental delivery, and during abruption.

- Dyspnoea
- Cyanosis
- Hypoxaemia
- Hypotension
- Cardiovascular collapse
- Convulsions
- Death: AFE carries 80% mortality, which occurs within the first hour

Management
- This is entirely supportive, and includes, as with all maternal catastrophes
- Immediate delivery of the foetus

Venous air embolus

Features
- During craniotomy, in 2–40%
- Sitting position
- Embolus ends in the right ventricle, where it may compromise cardiac output if large enough
- In cases of patent foramen ovale, a paradoxical embolus may occur with return of the embolus to vital tissue which will include the brain
- Nitrous oxide causes any air embolus to enlarge. The use of a stethoscope and a capnograph will allow early detection, with a 'mill wheel' murmur and a decrease in end-tidal CO_2

Management
- Stop any further embolism by flooding the operation site with saline and packs, and supporting the circulation with 100% oxygen and fluids. Compress neck veins to elevate CVP
- Left side down, elevate legs
- In some cases air may be retrieved from the right side of the heart if a central line is in place

Status asthmaticus

Recognition
- Dyspnoea (inability to speak is a grave sign)
- Cyanosis
- Reduced peak expiratory flow rate (PEFR) to less than 30% predicted
- Pulsus paradoxus, especially if more than 20 mmHg
- Arterial blood gas analysis showing reduced O_2, proceeding to hypercapnic (respiratory) acidosis

Beware: Silent chest, drowsy patient.

Management
- Oxygen
- Bronchodilators by infusion or nebuliser
- Hydrocortisone 4 mg/kg i.v.
- Antibiotics
- Ventilation if exhausted or if CO_2 accumulating

Status epilepticus

Recognition
- Tonic-clonic seizures
- Cyanosis if intercostals involved
- Tongue biting
- Incontinence

Management
- Protect from injury
- Diazemuls 5 mg/min until seizures controlled

Alternatives include general anaesthesia with thiopentone and a subsequent rapid intubation.

Epiglottitis

Recognition
- Stridor (but this is also seen in croup), and use of accessory muscles
- Severe systemic insult (which is not seen in croup)
- Child aged 3–5 (croup is seen between 6/12 and 3 y)

- Fever
- Drooling
- No coryzal signs (contrasting with croup)

Management
- Calm atmosphere; avoid moving the child, cannulation or examination; do not lie the child down
- Availability of emergency measures for airway control, i.e. tracheostomy
- Gaseous induction of anaesthesia, sitting
- Intubation; laryngeal opening is where it always is, behind the epiglottis, but the only clue may be bubbles from between the cords
- Antibiotics: Chloramphenicol and ampicillin
- Intubation with or without ventilation for 24 h

Total spinal anaesthesia

Recognition
- Rapidly ascending dense block following apparant epidural administration of local anaesthetic. It may also occur in regional blocks around the head and neck
- Inability to cough (inspiration is a diaphragmatic movement and thus an unreliable sign, whereas expiration is intercostal)
- Arm weakness
- Loss of consciousness
- Cardiovascular collapse as cardiac accelerator fibres (upper thoracic) are blocked, in addition to existing sympathetic block

Management
- Protect airway – intubation will be necessary, but first
- Administer 100% oxygen
- Elevate feet, uterine displacement in the obstetric patient if not delivered
- Rapid i.v. infusion
- Vasopressor – ephedrine 6 mg repeated until effect obtained
- Ensure prevention of awareness

Major haemorrhage

Recognition
- Tachycardia, which precedes
- Hypotension (unless cardiac drugs present)
- Pallor
- Sweating
- Cyanosis
- Hyperventilation
- Confusion
- Oliguria

Management
- Resuscitate – see introduction to this section
- Multiple wide-bore cannulation and infusion; blood, starches and colloid, all probably better than crystalloid
- Remember to send for the blood!
- Pneumatic anti-shock garments
- Correct acidosis, electrolyte disturbance and coagulation derangement, if present
- Inotropic support to prevent renal failure

Pneumothorax

Recognition
- Be aware of the risk in trauma, central cannulation, brachial plexus block, during positive pressure ventilation, emphysema, in Marfans and other tall young men
- Cyanosis, tachypnoea
- Assymetrical chest movement
- Tracheal deviation – away from the side of a tension pneumo-thorax, towards the side of a simple pneumothorax
- Tachycardia and hypotension
- Surgical Emphysema

Management
- Secure airway
- Discontinue nitrous oxide (if in use) and give 100% oxygen
- If under tension: 14 G cannula into 2nd intercostal space in mid-clavicular line, prior to
- Definitive intrapleural drainage

Awareness

Awareness is a major cause of litigation and is seen in paralysed patients (notably when using total intravenous anaesthesia) and obstetrics.

Recognition
- Pressure, rate, sweat and tears scale (PRST): Score less than 4 implies sleep
- Isolated forearm technique
- Skin conductance
- Lower oesophageal sphincter contractility
- Frontalis EMG
- EEG: Awake = low amplitude, high frequency asleep = high amplitude, low frequency
- Bispectral index
- Evoked responses: probably the way forward; auditory or visual

Management
- Avoid it: Use a volatile and a volatile monitor
- Ensure analgesia and patient safety
- Suspend surgery
- Full explanation to patient

Post-tonsillectomy haemorrhage

Recognition
- Irritable child in first 12 h post-tonsillectomy
- Hypovolaemia
- Occult bleeding, swallowed into stomach

Management
- Inhalational induction, or
- Rapid sequence induction: Either way anticipate difficulty and expect to use a smaller tube than at original operation
- Extubate awake and on side, head down. The child will vomit

Diabetic ketoacidosis

Recognition
- Reduced conscious level
- Ketones on breath and in urine
- Advanced dehydration
- Acidosis with increased anion gap

Management
- Insulin by infusion
- Correction of hypovolaemia with saline, not dextrose until blood glucose in normal range; up to 100 ml/kg may be required in the initial phase in extreme cases
- Attention to serum potassium which will fall with correction of glucose
- Use bicarbonate only in extreme cases

Addisonian crisis

Recognition
- Apathy, coma
- Hypoglycaemia
- Hyperkalaemia
- Trauma, infection, abrupt withdrawal of steroid therapy, Waterhouse-Friedrickson syndrome

Beware: Surgical and anaesthetic trauma in the long-term or recent short-term steroid user.

Management
- Correction of hypovolaemia
- Steroids; both glucocorticoid replacement (hydrocortisone) and mineralocorticoid replacement (fludrocortisone) will be needed
- Correction of hyperkalaemia and hyponatraemia

Pulmonary embolus

Recognition
- Dyspnoea, tachypnoea

- Cyanosis
- Circulatory collapse
- RH strain or S1Q3T3 on ECG
- ABG: $\downarrow O_2$ and $\downarrow CO_2$

Beware: 10th day postop total hip replacement

Management
- Anticoagulation, or in extreme cases
- Thrombolysis
- Analgesia
- Thoracotomy and embolectomy under bypass in refractory situations

Pyloric stenosis

Features
- Obstruction between stomach and duodenum and mismatched loss of electrolyte and buffer from those two sites
- The overriding need to conserve Na^+ in the kidneys which prevents correction of the problem
- So, while there is vomiting loss of K^+ and H^+, these ions are still excreted in the urine in order to maintain Na^+. The result of this is:
  - Hypochloraemic alkalosis
  - Hypokalaemia
  - Haemoconcentration

Management
- Achieve normovolaemia with saline, with potassium supplements. Use Cl^- as guide to success in correction of dehydration and acidosis
- Pass nasogastric tube
- Rapid sequence induction after aspiration of tube
- Extubate awake following NG aspiration
- Infiltrate wound with local anaesthetic
- Feed on 2nd day

INDEX